W9-CCE-981

Language and Motor Speech Disorders in Adults

Second Edition

Harvey Halpern

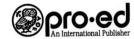

pro·ed
An International Publisher

8700 Shoal Creek Boulevard
Austin, Texas 78757-6897
800/897-3202   Fax 800/397-7633
Order online at http://www.proedinc.com

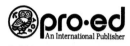

© 2000, 1986 by PRO-ED, Inc.
8700 Shoal Creek Boulevard
Austin, Texas 78757-6897
800/897-3202   Fax 800/397-7633
Order online at http://www.proedinc.com

The PRO-ED Studies in Communicative Disorders series
Series Editor: Harvey Halpern

Library of Congress Cataloging-in-Publication Data

Halpern, Harvey.
    Language and motor speech disorders in adults / Harvey Halpern.—
2nd ed.
        p.   cm.—(PRO-ED studies in communicative disorders)
    Includes bibliographical references and index.
    ISBN 0-89079-826-5 (alk. paper)
        1. Speech disorders.   2. Language disorders.   I. Title.
    II. Series.
RC423.H324   1999
616.85'5—dc21   99-32912
                                                                              CIP

This book is designed in Eras and Palatino.

Production Director: Alan Grimes
Production Coordinator: Dolly Fisk Jackson
Managing Editor: Chris Olson
Art Director: Thomas Barkley
Designer: Jason Crosier
Print Buyer: Alicia Woods
Preproduction Coordinator: Chris Anne Worsham
Staff Copyeditor: Martin Wilson
Project Editor: Jennifer Knoblock
Publishing Assistant: Jason Morris

Printed in the United States of America

1   2   3   4   5   6   7   8   9   10   04   03   02   01   00

This book is dedicated to Matthew, Lizzy, Kenny, Andrea, David, Annabelle, Juliet, Georgie, Maddy, and Jake.

Contents

Preface

This introductory book provides an overview of the major neurogenically caused speech and language disorders in adults. Chapter 1 provides some definitions used in speech, language, and cognition and introduces the six major disorders. Chapter 2 reviews the neural basis of speech and language and touches upon the speech and/or language impairment that results from damage to the neural system. Chapter 3 contains a discussion of the language disorder associated with adult aphasia. Chapter 4 addresses the communication disorders associated with right-hemisphere damage. Chapter 5 deals with the communication disorders associated with dementia. Chapter 6 presents the communication disorders associated with traumatic brain injury. Chapter 7 describes the motor speech disorders associated with dysarthria. Chapter 8 provides a discussion of the motor speech disorders associated with apraxia of speech.

Acknowledgments

I would like to give special thanks to the following individuals who made this manuscript possible. To the three readers who offered invaluable comments and suggestions: Dr. Joseph R. Duffy, Mayo Clinic, who read the early stages of this manuscript; Dr. Robert Goldfarb, Lehman College, who read the later stages of this manuscript; and Dr. Carole Ferrand, Hofstra University, who read the chapter devoted to the neural basis for speech and language.

To the people at PRO-ED: Dr. Donald D. Hammill, president, for running a first-rate organization; Mr. Steven C. Mathews, vice president, for handling all contractual matters in an expert manner; Dr. James R. Patton, executive editor, for graciously providing help, encouragement, and excellent advice on an almost 24-hour basis; Ms. Chris Anne Worsham, preproduction coordinator, for attending to all matters concerning the drawings and illustrations in a very fine professional manner; and Ms. Chris Olson, managing editor, for her patience during the final editing process.

To the late Dr. Fred Darley, professor emeritus, Mayo Foundation, for expanding my view of neurogenic communication disorders in adults, and to all my students and patients for providing the arena in which I learned a great deal of the subject matter.

CHAPTER 1

Introduction

The purpose of this book is to provide a clinically oriented, introductory framework for the major speech-language-communication disorders encountered by speech–language pathologists (SLPs) and other clinicians who work with adults with acquired neuropathologies. Specifically, this book will deal with the symptoms, etiology, diagnosis, and treatment of aphasia, the communication disorders associated with right-hemisphere damage, dementia, and traumatic brain injury (TBI), dysarthria, and apraxia of speech.

These communication disorders were chosen because they are the most frequent of the adult neuropathologies and because they resemble one another in certain features. It is important to differentiate these particular speech-language-communication disorders from one another because speech and/or language therapy might be similar, different, or not indicated at all.

Following are some definitions of terms that will be used throughout the book. They are presented, along with some of the characteristics typically associated with each of the communication disorders, for the purpose of showing some of the similarities and differences among the disorders.

Definitions

A *communication disorder* (American Speech-Language-Hearing Association [ASHA], 1993) is an impairment in the ability to receive, send, process, and comprehend concepts of verbal, nonverbal, and graphic symbol systems. It may be evident in the processes of hearing, language, and/or speech. It may range in severity from mild to profound. It may be developmental or acquired. Individuals may demonstrate one or any combination of communication disorders. The communication disorder may be a primary disability or it may be secondary to other disabilities.

A *speech disorder* (ASHA, 1993) is an impairment of the articulation of speech sounds, fluency, and/or voice. An *articulation disorder* is the atypical production of speech sounds characterized by substitutions, omissions, additions, or distortions that may interfere with intelligibility. A *fluency disorder* is an interruption in the flow of speaking characterized by atypical rate, rhythm, and repetitions in sounds, syllables, words, and phrases. This may be accompanied by excessive tension, struggle behavior, and secondary mannerisms. A *voice disorder* is characterized by the abnormal production and/or absence of vocal quality, pitch, loudness, resonance, and/or duration, which is inappropriate for an individual's age and/or sex.

A *language disorder* (ASHA, 1993) is impaired comprehension and/or use of spoken, written, and/or other symbol systems. The disorder may involve the form of language (phonology, morphology, syntax). *Phonology* is the sound system of a language and the rules that govern the sound combinations. *Morphology* is the system that governs the structure of words and the construction of word forms. *Syntax* is the system governing the order and combination of words to form sentences, and the relationships among the elements within a sentence.

The disorder may involve the content of language (semantics). *Semantics* is the system that governs the meanings of words and sentences. It must be noted that a disturbance in the semantic aspect of language is probably the most common error found in all of the neurogenic adult language disorders. The disorder may also involve the function of language (pragmatics). *Pragmatics* is the system that combines the above language components into functional and socially appropriate communication. Pragmatics (Prutting & Kirchner, 1987) would involve eye contact with the listener, topic maintenance, turn-taking, modulation of loudness, proper decorum in the communicative setting, facial and bodily gestures that reflect the mood, proper use of register, and providing relevant information to the listener.

Cognitive functioning involves orientation, arousal, attention, speed of processing, memory, abstract reasoning, and visuo–spatial perception. _Orientation_ is the ability to locate oneself in one's environment with reference to time (year, month, day, date, hour, etc.), place (where one thinks he is at the moment), and person (the identification of self and other people). _Arousal_ is an aspect of consciousness and is the next step above coma, which is a loss of consciousness.

Attention is attending to stimuli in space and the ability to hold objects, events, words, or thoughts in one's consciousness. _Selective attention_ is the ability to zero in on selected visual or auditory stimuli despite a host of other, competing stimuli. It is the ability to pick out the figure from the background and maintain attention to that figure long enough to complete a successful response. For example, if someone is shown a strongly limned picture of a sailboat (figure) to respond to but instead attends to some faintly drawn cloud in the distance (background) or to a number in the corner of the picture (background). (See Chapter 6 for a further discussion of attention.)

Speed of processing refers to the amount of time it takes for a person to absorb information. It is especially apparent under timed conditions. _Memory_ is the mental faculty or power that enables one to retain and to recall, through unconscious associative processes, previously experienced sensations, impressions, ideas, and concepts, and all information that has been consciously learned (Mosby Medical, Nursing, and Allied Health Dictionary, 1994). (See Chapters 5 and 6 for a further discussion of memory.)

Abstract reasoning is the process of looking at evidence, making inferences, and drawing conclusions. This reasoning allows one to draw inferences from experience and to find similarities among different but related phenomena (e.g., putting things in categories according to size, color, function, material, etc.). For example, someone looks at a picture of an old model "T" Ford and another picture of a 1999 Ford automobile and puts both pictures in the category called "cars," despite their obvious differences. Abstract reasoning is the ability to find the common thread (four wheels, a steering wheel, an area for the engine, an area for the driver and others, etc.) among things that appear superficially different.

Perception refers to the ability to organize incoming sensory stimuli by recognizing features and their relationships and then combining them with previous knowledge of these features (memory). Perception is the level above basic vision or hearing, and the level below reading or auditory comprehension. *Visuo–spatial perception* skills can include the ability to copy two- and three-dimensional drawings (e.g., circle, red cross, cube, cylinder, etc.), connect a series of numbers, draw on command a house or clock face, or reproduce figures that an examiner makes out of matches (Cummings and Benson, 1992).

Emotion includes mood and affect. Mood indicates the inner and subjective feelings of the patient, whereas affect is the outward expression of emotion. *Personality* is a third aspect of emotion, and refers to total behavior over time and to the person's immediate emotional state (Cummings & Benson, 1992).

Communication Disorders

The following communication disorders are discussed in this book.

Adult Aphasia

Adult aphasia typically has a sudden onset in middle and older age. The etiology is a brain lesion in the language-dominant hemisphere. The disorder is mostly chronic, with some cases of progressive aphasia. Typically, cognitive abilities are normal or near normal.

The impairment can range from mild to severe, but the language components are affected regardless of severity. In many cases, the language components are affected unevenly; that is, some components are better than others.

The language impairment does stand out in relation to other abilities. Generally, the phonologic, morphologic, syntactic, and semantic components can be affected, with the pragmatic component mostly intact. Personality and behavior are typically normal or near normal. Therapy mostly involves a language stimulation approach.

Communication Disorders Associated with Right-Hemisphere Damage

These disorders typically have a sudden onset in middle and older age. The etiology is a brain lesion in the right hemisphere (non-dominant for language). The disorder is mostly chronic. Cognitive abilities can be affected.

Language impairment, if present, is mostly in the mild range and does not stand out in relation to other abilities. The phonologic, morphologic, and syntactic components remain intact, while the semantic and pragmatic components may be affected. Personality and behavior may also be affected and can range from bizarre to near normal. Therapy mostly involves cognitive and executive planning approaches, with some language stimulation if needed.

Communication Disorders Associated with Dementia

These disorders typically have a gradual onset (although those accompanying vascular dementia can occur abruptly) in older age. The etiology is brain damage involving both hemispheres. The disorder is mostly progressive. Cognitive abilities are affected in direct proportion to the mild, moderate, and advanced stages of the disorder.

In *cortical dementia*, typically, the language components are affected according to the stage of the disorder. In the mild stage, the phonologic, morphologic, and syntactic components are all intact, while the semantic and pragmatic components begin to deteriorate. In the moderate stage, the phonologic component is intact, while the morphologic and syntactic components begin to deteriorate, and the semantic and pragmatic components further deteriorate. In the advanced stage, the phonologic component begins to deteriorate, along with a further deterioration of the morphologic and syntactic components, and a still greater deterioration of the semantic and pragmatic components. The language impairment does not stand out in relation to other abilities.

In *subcortical dementia*, typically there is no distinctive language breakdown. Language becomes restricted and simplified, and in the advanced stages there may be auditory comprehension and naming problems. Of the language components, the semantic and pragmatic aspects would most likely be affected. Speech can be dysarthric.

Personality and behavior are affected in both cortical and subcortical dementia. Therapy involves mostly cognitive approaches and, if necessary, the methods used for dysarthria.

Communication Disorders Associated with Traumatic Brain Injury

These disorders have a sudden onset and mostly appear in younger age (primarily in males) and in those over 75 years old. Typically, the etiology is brain damage involving both hemispheres. The disorder can be temporary or chronic. Cognitive abilities typically are affected in direct proportion to the severity of the disorder (mild, moderate, severe).

The language components are affected according to the stage of the disorder. In the mild stage, the phonologic, morphologic, and syntactic components are intact, but the semantic and pragmatic components may be impaired. In the moderate stage, the phonologic, morphologic, and syntactic components are intact, the semantic component may be impaired, and the pragmatic component is impaired. In the severe stage, the phonologic component remains intact, the morphologic and syntactic components may be impaired, and the semantic and pragmatic components are impaired.

The language impairment does not stand out in relation to other abilities. Personality and behavior are affected according to the severity of the disorder and can range from bizarre (severe stage) to near normal (mild stage). Therapy involves mostly cognitive and executive planning approaches.

Dysarthria

Dysarthria can have a sudden or gradual onset and can appear at any age. The etiology can be neurological impairment within the central nervous system (brain and spinal cord), or the peripheral nervous system (cranial nerves and spinal nerves). The site of lesion can be either focal, multifocal, or diffuse. The disorder can be temporary, chronic, or progressive. Typically, cognitive abilities are normal or near normal.

Dysarthria is a motor speech disorder involving motor execution problems within the neuromuscular system, and should present no language impairment. The affected speech components can involve respiration, phonation, resonation, articulation, and prosody in any combination. Personality and behavior are mostly normal or near normal. Therapy involves the reestablishment of the neuromuscular system's motor execution capabilities in the presence of an intact motor programming component.

Apraxia of Speech

Apraxia of speech typically has a sudden onset in middle and older age. The etiology is a brain lesion in the language-dominant hemisphere (focal). The disorder is mostly chronic. Typically, cognitive abilities are normal or near normal.

Apraxia of speech is a motor speech disorder involving programming problems within the neuromuscular system, and should present no language impairment. However, if accompanied by aphasia, as it often is, language will be impaired. The affected speech components involve articulation and prosody. Personality and behavior are mostly normal or near normal. Therapy involves the reestablishment of the neuromuscular system's motor programming capabilities in the presence of an intact motor execution component.

CHAPTER 2

The Neural Basis of Speech and Language

Introduction

This section gives the reader a brief overview of what takes place neurally when a person starts a conversation by saying, "Hello. How are you? How was your vacation trip?" to another individual whom he or she meets on the street. Simply put, the steps involved would be as follows:

1. basic vision—seeing a person on the street

2. visual perception—recognizing the person as someone the speaker knows

3. cognition—the desire to speak with this person about a trip that the speaker may want to take in the future

4. language—searching for the right sounds, syllables, words, and sentences, all presented in the right order, with meaning properly related to the greeting and the subject matter, to be expressed with a positive attitude

5. motor programming or planning—readying the speech mechanism just prior to speaking so that the production is correct

6. motor production or execution—speaking

7. feedback—(a) from self: hearing and feeling oneself speak and then using that information as a guide for further appropriate speaking (e.g., usually we know when something said doesn't sound right, and we either repeat it or put it in different words); (b) from others: looking at and listening to another person speak to help determine what to say next (e.g., responding to questions from someone who looks and sounds angry as opposed to someone who doesn't).

Responding to auditory feedback from oneself or from others involves the hearing of sound (basic hearing). Recognizing that sound as speech and not some other environmental noise is auditory perception. Understanding what is said is language comprehension. All of the steps mentioned above, with the exception of cognition, will be commented on in the neural outline that follows. The neural basis for cognition (thinking and behavior) probably involves bilateral cortical areas (especially the frontal lobes) as the prime movers, assisted by subcortical and brain stem systems. Because of the widespread neural activity, localization of cognitive functions is quite difficult. However, cognition and defects of cognition are noted in other parts of this manuscript (e.g., the chapters dealing with right hemisphere damage, dementia, and traumatic brain injury).

The information in the following outline has been gleaned from Duffy (1995), Kent (1997), Love and Webb (1996), Webster (1999), and Zemlin (1998); the organization of the outline mostly follows that of Love and Webb. The reader is referred to these sources for further elaboration of any of the topics mentioned in the outline. In a number of places within the outline, examples are given of the speech and/or language problem that can occur if there is damage to certain portions of the neural system. Most of the speech and/or language problems given as examples are mentioned further in other parts of this manuscript.

The Neuron

The neuron, or nerve cell, consists of a cell body, dendrites, and an axon (Figure 2.1). The *cell body* (intracellular) contains a high concentration of potassium and low concentrations of sodium and chloride, compared to the fluids outside the cell body (extracellular). The concentrations are

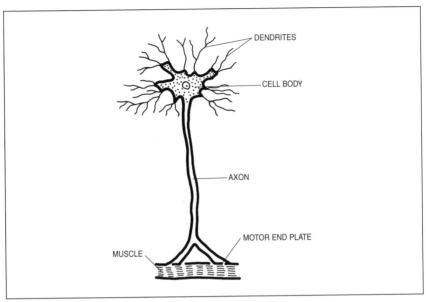

Figure 2.1. A neuron, with its cell body, dendrites, and axon, synapsing at the myoneural junction of the muscle.

reversed in the extracellular fluids, thus creating an electrical current or transmission of neural impulse. *Dendrites* are numerous short projections that carry neural impulses to the cell body. The *axon* carries neural impulses away from the cell body. The neuron can transmit neural impulses to other neurons, glands, or muscles.

The juncture at which neural impulses are transmitted is called a *synapse*; neurochemical transmitters aid in moving the neural impulses along. *Myelin*, a fatty sheath that insulates the larger axons, is said to increase the speed of neural transmission and also to reduce interference with the neural message. There may be about 100 billion neurons in the human nervous system. Axons can produce anywhere from 1,000 to 10,000 synapses, and their cell bodies and dendrites receive neural data from about 1,000 other neurons. As a result, the number of synapses occurring in the brain may be about 100 trillion.

The Human Nervous System

The human nervous system is made up of the central, peripheral, and autonomic nervous systems. The areas of the human nervous system that will be reviewed in the following pages are those that are vital for speech and language. The *central nervous system* (CNS) contains the brain, spinal cord, meninges, ventricles, and blood supply. The *peripheral nervous system* (PNS) is composed of the spinal peripheral nerves and the cranial nerves (Figure 2.2). The *autonomic nervous system* (ANS) contains a sympathetic division and a parasympathetic division.

The Central Nervous System

The central nervous system (CNS) consists of the brain, spinal cord, meninges, ventricles, and blood supply.

The Brain

The brain is composed of the cerebral hemispheres, the basal ganglia, the cerebellum, and the brain stem. The largest part of the brain is called the *cerebrum* and is made up of the two cerebral hemispheres and the basal ganglia. The cerebral cortex covers the cerebrum and is composed

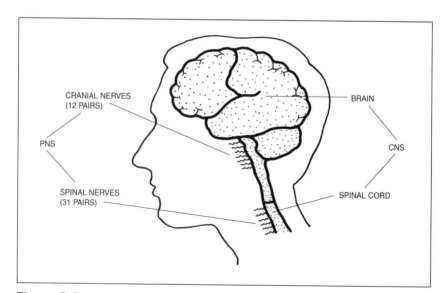

Figure 2.2. The CNS (brain and spinal cord) and PNS (12 pairs of cranial nerves and 31 pairs of spinal nerves).

of many prominent sulci or fissures (grooves on the surface of the brain or spinal cord) and gyri (elevations or ridges on the surface of the cerebrum).

Cerebral Hemispheres

The cerebral hemispheres are composed of a left and a right hemisphere and are connected by a mass of white matter called the *corpus callosum*. The purpose of the corpus callosum is to pass neuronal information from one hemisphere to the other. Medically directed severance of the corpus callosum has led to a good deal of "split brain" research. Included in the findings of this research is the observation that the left hemisphere serves a different purpose than the right hemisphere. Some of the functions of the left hemisphere are involvement in language and analytical and logical aspects, whereas the right hemisphere is involved with perceptual, spatial, intuitive, and holistic aspects (e.g., a lesion in a language area of the left hemisphere can result in aphasia, whereas a lesion in the right hemisphere can result in the patient's inability to draw information through inference that is arrived at by taking a holistic and intuitive approach).

The *longitudinal cerebral fissure,* which runs from the front to the back of the brain, separates the two hemispheres (Figure 2.3). The cerebral cortex in each hemisphere is partitioned into the frontal, parietal, temporal, and occipital lobes (Figure 2.4). Lying beneath the outer surface of the cerebral cortex is a fifth lobe called the limbic lobe.

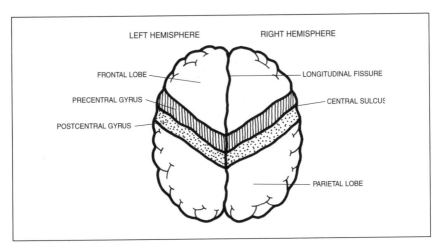

Figure 2.3. A superior view of the cerebral hemispheres.

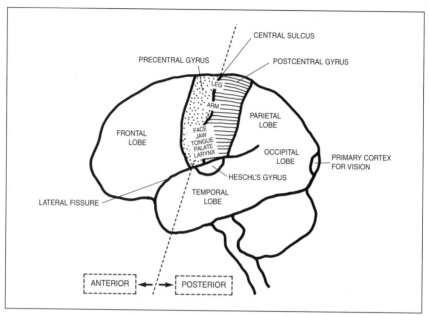

Figure 2.4. Lateral view showing the location of the four lobes of the brain.

The frontal lobe. The frontal lobe is bounded in the back by the *central sulcus* and below by the *lateral fissure.* The brain is divided into anterior and posterior regions by the central sulcus. Within the frontal lobe is the *precentral gyrus,* which lies immediately anterior to the central sulcus. The precentral gyrus is also known as the primary motor cortex or "motor strip" area, and it controls voluntary muscular movement on the opposite side of the body (Figure 2.4).

The neurons within the primary motor cortex are organized in a pattern of a person ("homunculus" or little man) standing upside down. Neurons devoted to motor movements in the face and neck area are closest to the lateral fissure, and neurons devoted to motor movements of the toes and leg are closest to the longitudinal cerebral fissure (Figure 2.4). Some parts of the body require fine motor movement, whereas other parts require less precise motor movement. There is a greater array of neurons devoted to the small muscles of the larynx, palate, tongue, jaw, and face than to the arm or leg. The number of neurons allocated for voluntary movement of a body part is typically not commensurate with its size. A lesion in the primary motor cortex within areas involving movements of the lips, tongue, or larynx can result in certain types of dysarthria.

Located in front of the precentral gyrus are the *premotor* and *supplementary motor areas* (Figure 2.5). These areas receive information from other regions of the brain, and their purpose is to integrate, refine, and plan or program motor speech output (e.g., a lesion in the premotor areas can result in certain types of dysarthria, or if in the dominant hemisphere, an apraxia of speech). *Broca's area* is in the third frontal gyrus of the dominant hemisphere (Figure 2.5). This important area plays a main role in motor speech programming and also connects to other parts of the brain involved with speech and language (e.g., a lesion in Broca's area can result in apraxia of speech).

The parietal lobe. The parietal lobe is bounded in the front by the central sulcus and below by the back end of the lateral fissure. Within the parietal lobe is the *postcentral gyrus,* which is located in back of the central sulcus (Figure 2.4). The postcentral gyrus is a mirror image to the "motor strip" area of the frontal lobe and is a primary sensory cortical area ("sensory strip") having to do with temperature, pain, touch, and proprioception.

Proprioception (includes the senses of movement, vibration, pressure, position, equilibrium, and deep pain) enables one to realize exactly where the individual parts of the body are in space, and the rela-

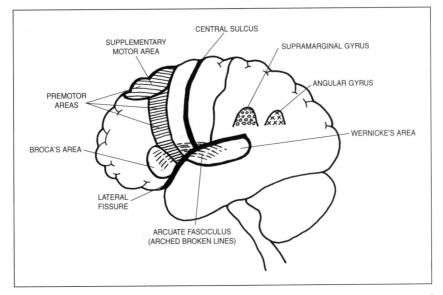

Figure 2.5. Lateral view of the left (dominant) hemisphere, showing the location of the language and motor speech programming (or planning) areas.

tionship of one body part to another (e.g., tongue in relation to the alveolar ridge in the production of lingua–alveolar sounds). This somatosensory cortex in the dominant hemisphere appears to play a part in motor speech programming, especially in the integration of sensory information in preparation for motor activity (e.g., a lesion in this area can result in apraxia of speech).

The parietal lobe in the dominant hemisphere also contains the supramarginal gyrus and the angular gyrus (Figure 2.5). The *supramarginal gyrus* curves around the back end of the lateral fissure and is responsible for the formulation of written language and possibly for phonological storage (e.g., a lesion in this area can result in aphasia). The *angular gyrus* lies directly behind the supramarginal gyrus and plays a major role in reading comprehension (e.g., a lesion in this area can result in aphasia).

The temporal lobe. The temporal lobe is bounded on top by the lateral fissure and in the back by the front border of the occipital lobe. Three important areas in the temporal lobe of the dominant hemisphere are *Heschl's gyrus*, *Wernicke's area*, and the *insula* (or the Island of Reil). Heschl's gyrus (or primary auditory cortex) is located on the lateral fissure, two thirds of the way back on the upper surface of the temporal lobe (Figure 2.4). It is the cortical center for hearing, responsible for appreciating the meaning of sound (e.g., a lesion in this area can result in auditory processing problems, which can lead to auditory comprehension deficit). Wernicke's area (an auditory association area) is located on the back part of the superior temporal gyrus (Figure 2.5) and plays a major role in auditory comprehension and other language abilities (e.g., a lesion in this area can result in aphasia). The insula, which can be seen if the two borders of the lateral fissure are pulled apart, is in the paralimbic area. The function of the insula is not clearly defined, but a lesion there can result in aphasia or apraxia of speech.

The occipital lobe. The occipital lobe is located at the back of the cerebral hemisphere. It is bounded in the front by the parietal and temporal lobes and in back by the longitudinal fissure. The *primary visual cortex* and *visual association areas* are situated in the occipital lobe. The primary visual cortex (Figure 2.4) is responsible for basic vision (e.g., a lesion in this area can produce degrees of blindness). The visual association area is needed for integrating and organizing incoming visual stimuli (e.g., a lesion here can result in visual perception problems, which in turn can influence reading comprehension).

The limbic lobe. The limbic lobe is situated on the medial surface of the cortex and contains the orbital frontal region, the cingulate gyrus, and the medial portions of the temporal lobe. The limbic system regulates emotions and behavior (e.g., a lesion in this system can affect prosody, or possibly pragmatic abilities).

The association areas. As mentioned previously, there are primary centers for motor, sensory, hearing, and visual functioning. These centers are connected to one another and to other parts of the brain by association areas. The association areas are responsible for higher mental functioning, including language, and are located in the lobes of each hemisphere.

The *frontal association area* is responsible for initiation and integration of purposeful behavior and for planning and carrying out sequences of volitional movement. The *parietal association area* or *somesthetic area* is responsible for the discrimination and integration of tactile information. The *temporal* or *auditory association area* is needed for the discrimination and integration of auditory information. The *visual association area* is responsible for the discrimination and integration of visual information. A lesion in an association area of the dominant hemisphere can result in aphasia; or a lesion in a pathway connecting one association area with another can result in aphasia, as in the case of the *arcuate fasciculus* (Figure 2.5), which connects the association area of the temporal lobe with that of the frontal lobe.

The Basal Ganglia (or Basal Nuclei)

In another part of the brain are subcortical structures called the basal ganglia. They are a mass of gray matter that lies deep within the cerebrum and below the cerebral cortex. The basal ganglia consist of the caudate nucleus, the globus pallidus, and the putamen; grouped together, these are called the *corpus striatum* (Figure 2.6). The globus pallidus and putamen are sometimes named together as the *lentiform nucleus.* The basal ganglia are responsible for controlling and stabilizing motor functions and for interpreting sensory information so as to guide and influence motor behavior (e.g., a lesion in the basal ganglia can result in dysarthria).

The Cerebellum

The cerebellum is located just behind the pons and the medulla at the base of the occipital lobe (Figure 2.6). The cerebellum contains a right and left hemisphere that are connected by the *vermis* between the two hemispheres (Figure 2.7). These are the areas most involved in speech control. The cerebellum does not initiate motor movements, but through its connections to the spinal cord, cerebrum, pons, and medulla, it helps in coordinating the skilled, voluntary muscle activity

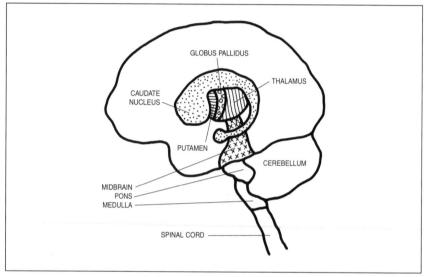

Figure 2.6. A sagittal section of the brain that shows the location of the spinal cord, brain stem (medulla, pons, midbrain, thalamus), basal ganglia (caudate nucleus, globus pallidus, putamen), and cerebellum. A sagittal section is a vertical cut or slice which divides the body into right and left halves, producing two equal, mirror-image parts.

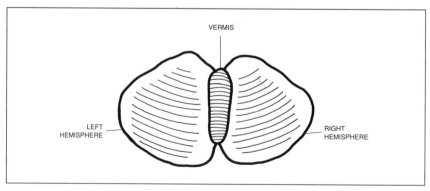

Figure 2.7. A superior view of the cerebellum showing the two hemispheres and the vermis.

produced elsewhere (e.g., a lesion in the cerebellum can result in dysarthria).

The Brain Stem

The brain also contains the brain stem, which appears as an upward extension of the spinal cord and thrusts upward into the brain between the cerebral hemispheres. In ascending order from the spinal cord, the brain stem consists of the medulla oblongata, the pons, the midbrain (mesencephalon), and two structures (diencephalon) called the thalamus and hypothalamus (Figure 2.6). Some authors include the thalamus and hypothalamus as part of the cerebrum.

The medulla and pons. The medulla contains nuclei for several of the cranial nerves, and ascending and descending tracts to and from the cortex that are important for the control of speech production. The pons contains nuclei for several of the cranial nerves, has major connections to the cerebellum, and has other connections to the cortex that are important for speech production (e.g., a lesion in a cranial nerve important for speech can result in dysarthria).

The midbrain, thalamus, and hypothalamus. The midbrain serves as a way station in the auditory and visual nervous systems, and contains the *substantia nigra.* The substantia nigra is responsible for the production of a chemical neurotransmitter named dopamine, which aids in motor control and muscle tone (e.g., a lesion in the substantia nigra can result in dysarthria).

The thalamus serves as a relay station for sensory information going to and from the sensory areas of the cortex, and has direct ties to cortical language and motor speech systems (Figure 2.6) (e.g., a lesion in the thalamus can result in aphasia). The hypothalamus controls aspects of emotional behavior (rage and aggression) and aids in the regulation of body temperature, food and water intake, and sexual and sleep behavior.

The Spinal Cord

In addition to the brain, the CNS also contains the spinal cord. The spinal cord extends from the skull through a large opening called the *foramen magnum* down to the lower back. The foramen magnum is the boundary between the medulla and the spinal cord. The spinal cord is encased in the vertebral column. A cross section of the spinal cord shows an *H*-shaped area of gray matter in the core of the spinal segment. The gray matter of the *H* shape contains motor and sensory neurons. The ventral or anterior portion of the cord conducts motor neurons, and the dorsal or posterior portion of the cord conducts sensory neurons.

The Spinal Nerves

Thirty-one pairs of spinal nerves (which along with the cranial nerves are part of the PNS) are attached to the spinal cord (Figure 2.2). The spinal cord, through these 31 pairs of nerves, relays sensory information from the receptor (e.g., skin) to the cortex for evaluation of the sensations of pain, temperature, touch, and vibration. The spinal nerves relay motor information from the CNS to the effector (e.g., muscles).

As with the cortex, the spinal cord contains gray and white matter. The gray matter contains the nerve cell bodies, and the white matter contains the ascending and descending nerve axon fibers. *Ascending tracts* carry sensory or afferent information, whereas *descending tracts* carry motor or efferent information.

The Reflex Arc

Occasionally, a motor response can avoid going through the higher centers of the cortex for interpretation; this shortcut is known as the reflex arc (Figure 2.8). For example, a receptor (e.g., skin) responds to pain or temperature and sends this information through an afferent (or sen-

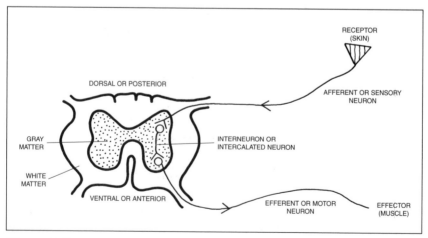

Figure 2.8. Cross section of the spinal cord showing the reflex arc.

sory) neuron, which sends it to the dorsal (or posterior) horn (within the *H* shape) within the spinal cord. At this point, instead of ascending to higher centers of the cortex, the impulse travels through an interneuron (or intercalated neuron) within the spinal cord to the ventral (or anterior) horn (within the *H* shape). From there, the impulse descends through an efferent (or motor) neuron and into the effector (e.g., muscles) whose action will cause a hand to be removed instantaneously and without thinking from water that is too hot. This is a simplified version of a reflex arc taking place at the spinal cord level. There are different types of reflexes that can take place at different levels within the nervous system.

The Meninges

The brain and the spinal cord are protected and nourished by a system involving the meninges, ventricles, and blood supply. Protection of the brain and spinal cord starts with the *hard bone* of the cranium and the *bony vertebral column* of the spinal cord. Below the bone are three membranes called the meninges (Figure 2.9). In descending order the meninges are composed of the *dura mater* ("tough mother"), *arachnoid mater* ("spider mother"), and *pia mater* ("delicate mother").

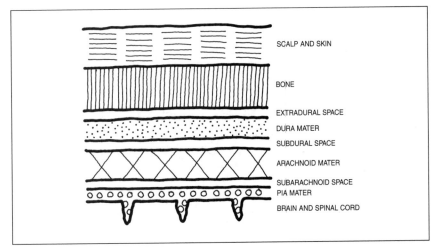

Figure 2.9. The meninges that cover the brain and the spinal cord.

There are several spaces that separate the meninges and provide a cushioning effect. Located between the outer bone and the dura mater is the *extradural space.* Located beneath the dura mater is the *subdural space.* Situated between the arachnoid mater and the pia mater is the *subarachnoid space,* which contains cerebrospinal fluid. (Physical trauma to the brain that tears or lacerates the meninges is identified as open head injury, and can affect speech, language, or cognition.)

The Ventricles

There is a network of cavities within the brain called ventricles that are connected to one another by small canals and ducts (Figure 2.10). Cerebrospinal fluid, which is produced by the choroid plexus within each ventricle, fills all the ventricles. Through small openings in particular ventricles, cerebrospinal fluid fills the subarachnoid space of the meninges. The cerebrospinal fluid aids in the nourishment of nerve tissues, regulates intracranial pressure, removes waste products, and

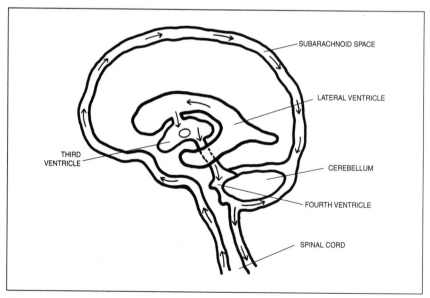

Figure 2.10. The ventricular system.

along with the meninges, cushions and protects the brain and spinal cord from physical trauma.

The ventricles involved are the *lateral ventricle*, the *third ventricle*, and the *fourth ventricle*. The lateral ventricle, which is paired (one in each hemisphere), is connected to the third ventricle through an opening called the intraventricular foramen (or the foramen of Monro). The third ventricle is connected to the fourth ventricle through the cerebral aqueduct (or the aqueduct of Sylvius). The fourth ventricle leads into the subarachnoid space through the foramen of Luschka and the foramen of Magendi. Through this ventricular route, the cerebrospinal fluid flows into the brain and the spinal cord.

The Blood Supply

Blood is composed of a liquid component called plasma, and solid components made up primarily of red corpuscles, white corpuscles, and platelets. Red corpuscles, which are produced in the bone marrow, are the cells that carry oxygen from the lungs to other parts of the body. The brain needs oxygen and other elements carried by the blood for its proper nutrition and functioning. If the blood supply to the brain is stopped for 5 minutes or longer, cell death can occur.

Arteries carry blood away from the heart, veins carry blood toward the heart, and capillaries connect the arteries to the veins. The blood supply to the brain is as follows (Figure 2.11): The heart pumps blood into the aorta (major artery), which then branches off into four main arteries called the two common carotid arteries (one for the left side and one for the right side) and the two common subclavian arteries (one for each side). The two common carotid arteries ascend into the brain, where they divide into an internal carotid artery and an external carotid artery on each side. The *external carotid branch* feeds the face area and is relatively unimportant for this review. The *internal carotid branch* further divides into the anterior and middle cerebral arteries (Figure 2.12). The *anterior cerebral artery* supplies the superior and anterior frontal lobes, corpus callosum, the medial surfaces of the hemispheres, and portions of the subcortical areas. The *middle cerebral artery* supplies most of the lateral surfaces of the hemispheres and portions of the subcortical areas.

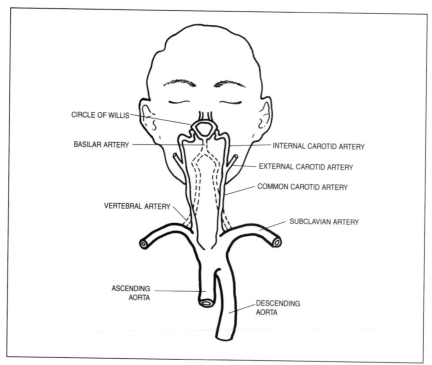

Figure 2.11. The major arteries supplying blood to the brain.

The two *common subclavian arteries* have branches called the vertebral arteries, which ascend into the brain. The *vertebral artery branches* (one from each side) join together to form the *basilar artery*. The basilar artery then ascends and divides into two *posterior cerebral arteries* (one for each hemisphere) (Figure 2.12), which supply the inferior lateral surface of the temporal lobe, and the lateral and medial surfaces of the occipital lobe. Through its branches, the basilar artery also supplies portions of the spinal cord, medulla, pons, midbrain, and cerebellum.

The circle of Willis (Figure 2.11) is formed in the brain stem by the joining together of the two internal carotid arteries and the two vertebral arteries. An interruption of the blood supply below the circle of Willis may not cause as much brain damage as lesions above the circle. The reason is that other undamaged blood channels can be utilized to feed all of the arteries below the circle. If an interruption occurs above the circle, alternative blood channels are not as readily available, and

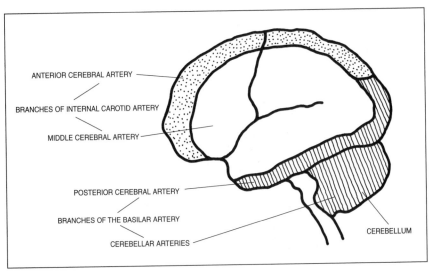

Figure 2.12. Lateral view of the left hemisphere showing the location of the anterior, middle, and posterior cerebral arteries.

this can lead to more severe problems (e.g., a cerebrovascular accident above the circle of Willis in the middle cerebral artery can result in aphasia).

The Motor System for Speech

The neural motor pathways for the control of speech reside at all levels of the human nervous system and consist of the pyramidal system and the extrapyramidal system. The pyramidal system (or direct motor system) contains the corticospinal tract and the corticobulbar tract; both tracts are responsible for skilled voluntary motor movement (Figure 2.13). The function of the pyramidal system is primarily facilitative.

The Corticospinal Tract
The corticospinal tract, which controls skilled voluntary movements of the limbs and trunk, begins in the motor cortex or in the premotor cortex, which is a depository for information coming from various cortical

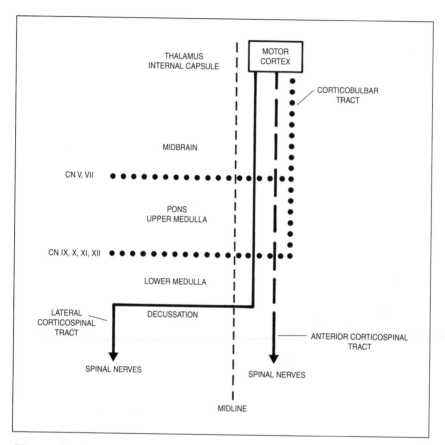

Figure 2.13. A schematic drawing of the pyramidal system in speech production, and the concept of the upper motor neuron (UMN) and the lower motor neuron (LMN). The pyramidal system (corticospinal and corticobulbar tracts) makes up the UMN. The cranial nerves (responsible for the innervation of the muscles used in phonation, resonance, and articulation) and the spinal nerves (responsible for the innervation of the muscles used in respiration) make up the LMN. CN = cranial nerve.

and subcortical locations. The area primarily involved is the precentral gyrus (motor strip area) of the frontal lobe (Figure 2.4) and to a lesser degree, the premotor area of the frontal lobe (Figure 2.5) and the postcentral gyrus (sensory strip area) of the parietal lobe (Figure 2.4).

The bilateral corticospinal tracts (Figure 2.13) descend from the cortex to a subcortical structure called the internal capsule, where they all converge. From the internal capsule, the tracts descend through the midbrain, the pons, the medulla, and then to various levels of the spinal cord, where they synapse with the spinal nerves of the peripheral nervous system.

Before reaching the spinal nerves, about 85% to 90% of the corticospinal tracts cross over (decussate) to the other side of the body in a structure named the upper medullary pyramids (hence the name *pyramidal system*). (A lesion above the crossover decussation point of the medullary pyramids can result in paralysis of a limb that is contralateral [opposite side] to the site of the lesion. A lesion below the crossover point can result in paralysis of a limb ipsilateral [same side] to the site of the lesion.) The 85% to 90% of the corticospinal tracts that do cross over are called the lateral corticospinal tracts, and the 10% to 15% that do not cross over are called the anterior corticospinal tracts.

The Corticobulbar Tract

The corticobulbar (bulbar, meaning "shaped like a bulb" is the old name for the medulla) tract controls the skilled voluntary movements of the speech muscles (except those used for respiration). The tract begins in the same area as the corticospinal tract and descends to the motor nuclei of the cranial nerves, which are located in the pons and the medulla (Figure 2.13). The corticobulbar tract has many ipsilateral and contralateral fibers, with crossover taking place at various levels of the brain stem. Because of the bilateral innervation that the corticobulbar tract produces, the majority of the midline structures work in bilateral symmetry (e.g., a unilateral lesion to the corticobulbar tract can result in a mild dysarthria because of help from the intact muscles of the other side).

The Extrapyramidal System

The extrapyramidal system (or indirect motor system) is made up of two major components—the indirect activation pathway and the control circuit areas.

The Indirect Activation Pathway

The indirect activation pathway (Duffy, 1995) consists of several short pathways that begin in the cerebral cortex and, through its connections, end in the spinal cord and in the cranial nerves. The indirect activation pathway is influenced by the basal ganglia and cerebellar control circuits, and through much of its journey intermingles with the corticospinal and corticobulbar tracts of the pyramidal system. Its influence on the spinal nerves is more certain than its influence on the cranial nerves.

The function of the indirect activation pathway (Duffy, 1995) is that it helps regulate reflexes and maintain posture, tone, and other associated activities. This helps the direct motor system in accomplishing the appropriate speed, range, and direction of specific muscular movements (e.g., a unilateral lesion in the indirect activation pathway can result in a unilateral upper motor neuron dysarthria; bilateral lesions can result in a spastic dysarthria). The indirect activation pathway contains many tracts that are inhibitive in function.

The Control Circuits

The control circuits consist of the *basal ganglia control circuit* and the *cerebellar control circuit* (Figure 2.6). These control circuits do not have direct contact with the cranial nerve nuclei and the spinal cord, but rather have contact with the cortex, with portions of the pyramidal system and indirect activation pathways, and with themselves. The function of the control circuits is to provide information and sensory feedback to the pyramidal system and indirect activation pathways about the posture, orientation in space, tone, and physical environment in which timed and coordinated muscular movement will take place.

Motor disturbances associated with the basal ganglia control circuit are typically called dyskinesias, which means involuntary movement disorders. Within the dyskinesias are hypokinesia, which means too little movement (e.g., symptoms shown in hypokinetic dysarthria), and hyperkinesia, which means too much movement (e.g., symptoms shown in hyperkinetic dysarthria).

Motor disturbances associated with the cerebellar control circuit are incoordination and hypotonia (a decrease in resistance when passive movement is performed) of muscular movements (e.g., a lesion in the cerebellar control circuit can result in ataxic dysarthria).

The Upper and Lower Motor Neuron

The Upper Motor Neuron

The upper motor neuron (UMN) pathways consist of the pyramidal system (or direct motor system), and a portion of the extrapyramidal system (or indirect motor system).

The pyramidal system contains the corticospinal tracts, which send motor impulses from the cortex to the spinal cord, and the corticobulbar tracts, which send motor impulses from the cortex to the cranial nerves located in the pons and the medulla (Figure 2.13). The portion of the extrapyramidal system that is a part of the UMN is the indirect activation pathway. The indirect activation pathway sends motor impulses from the cortex to the spinal cord, from the cortex to the cranial nerves, and from the cortex to the corticospinal and corticobulbar tracts.

The indirect activation pathway (Duffy, 1995) as part of the UMN (tracts that have direct input to the spinal nerves and the cranial nerves) is debatable because its anatomy and function are difficult to separate from the basal ganglia and cerebellar control circuits, and its input to the cranial nerves used for speech production is poorly understood. The control circuits do not have direct input to the spinal and cranial nerves, whereas the corticospinal, corticobulbar, and indirect activation tracts do have direct input.

The UMN pathways are contained in the CNS, and their function is to activate the lower motor neuron (LMN). Damage to the UMN can result in a *spastic paralysis*, which is primarily characterized by hypertonia (extreme tension of the muscles), hyperreflexia (an exaggeration of deep tendon reflexes), little or no atrophy (loss of bulk) of the musculature, and no fasciculations (fine muscle twitches). These characteristics can lead to decreased skilled movements, weakness, slowness, and reduced range of movement of the speech musculature (e.g., bilateral UMN damage can result in a spastic dysarthria).

The Lower Motor Neuron

The lower motor neuron (LMN) consists of the 31 pairs of spinal nerves and the 12 pairs of cranial nerves (Figure 2.2). The LMN pathways are activated by the UMN pathways, and then send motor impulses to the muscles for movement. The spinal nerves send motor impulses to the limbs, trunk, and the muscles used for respiration. The cranial nerves send motor impulses to the muscles of the speech mechanism (except those used for respiration).

Another name for the LMN is the final common pathway (FCP) because all motor activity must pass through it en route to the musculature. Damage to the LMN can result in a *flaccid paralysis*, which is primarily characterized by hypotonia, hyporeflexia, atrophy of the musculature, and fasciculations. Those characteristics can lead to weakness of the speech musculature. Lesions to the motor unit (Figure 2.14) of the LMN (spinal and cranial nerves) can occur in the cell body, in the axon leading to the muscle, at the neuromuscular junction, or in the muscle itself (e.g., bilateral damage to any portion of the motor unit can result in a flaccid dysarthria).

The Peripheral Nervous System

The peripheral nervous system (PNS) is composed of 31 pairs of spinal nerves and 12 pairs of cranial nerves (Figure 2.2).

The Spinal Nerves

The 31 pairs of spinal nerves leave the spinal cord and conduct sensory and motor impulses (functions) to and from other parts of the body (viscera, blood vessels, glands, and muscles). The spinal nerves (each pair) contain a *dorsal (posterior) root,* which carries sensory messages through afferent fibers to the CNS, and a *ventral (anterior) root,* which carries motor messages through efferent fibers from the CNS.

The *sensory messages* (e.g., pain, touch, temperature) are passed to the thalamus, which in turn sends the messages to the sensory cortex (postcentral gyrus) for evaluation. The *motor messages* are sent from the CNS (corticospinal tracts) to the spinal nerves of the PNS, which in turn send the message to the muscles of the limbs and the trunk.

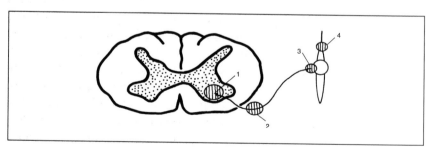

Figure 2.14. Lesion sites in the motor unit of the lower motor neuron: Site 1, cell body (motor neuron disease); site 2, axon (motor neuropathy); site 3, myoneural juncture (neuromyopathy); and site 4, muscle fiber (myopathy or dystrophy).

In descending order, the 31 pairs of spinal nerves consist of 8 pairs of cervical nerves, 12 pairs of thoracic nerves, 5 pairs of lumbar nerves, 5 pairs of sacral nerves, and 1 pair of coccygeal nerves. Portions of the thoracic division are responsible for the abdominal and intercostal muscles, and portions of the cervical division form the phrenic nerves, which are responsible for the very important diaphragm muscle. All of these muscles are involved in the respiratory component of speech production (e.g., bilateral lesions that produce significant weakness of the respiratory muscles can result in reduced loudness and reduced pitch variability, and can indirectly affect phonation [compensatory strained voice] and prosody [short phrases]).

The Cranial Nerves

There are 12 pairs of cranial nerves (one nerve of each pair on each side), although only the 7 pairs of cranial nerves most relevant for speech and hearing will be mentioned here. The 7 cranial nerves involved leave the pons or the medulla and conduct sensory and/or motor impulses to and from the periphery and the CNS. Motor messages are sent from the CNS (corticobulbar tracts) to the cranial nerve nuclei located in the pons and the medulla, and then out to the musculature of the speech mechanism and other portions of the head, neck, shoulders, and the abdominal and thoracic viscera.

Sensory messages come from the periphery and go to the cranial nerve nuclei located in the pons and the medulla, from where they are forwarded to the thalamus. In turn, the thalamus sends the messages to the sensory cortex (postcentral gyrus) for evaluation. Of the 7 cranial nerves most relevant for speech and hearing, only the cranial nerve responsible for hearing and balance does not follow this sensory route. The route for hearing and balance will be mentioned in another section.

Most of the cranial nerves receive bilateral neural innervation, some receive unilateral neural innervation, and some receive a mixture of bilateral and unilateral neural innervation (depending upon the branches of the cranial nerve) from the corticobulbar tract of the CNS.

A unilateral lesion affecting a cranial nerve receiving bilateral neural innervation will cause less severe speech problems than one receiving unilateral neural innervation. With bilateral tracts, the undamaged tract can compensate for the damaged one. Bilateral damage to bilateral tracts, and unilateral damage to unilateral tracts will produce more severe speech problems.

Below is a brief outline of the cranial nerves (CN) most relevant to speech production and hearing. Unless specified otherwise, sensory refers to the sensation of pain, touch, temperature, or vibration.

1. *Trigeminal* (CN V) receives sensory impulses from the jaw, lips, face, and tongue, and sends motor impulses to the jaw. Bilateral damage to the sensory function and/or the motor function can affect articulation and prosody (slow rate).

2. Facial (CN VII) receives sensory impulses from the anterior two thirds of the tongue (taste), soft palate (taste), and nasopharynx (taste), and sends motor impulses to the face, lips, and the stapedius muscle of the middle ear. Unilateral damage to the motor function can affect articulation (mild), and bilateral damage to the motor function can affect articulation (moderate to severe), prosody (slow rate), and facial expression (pragmatics?).

3. *Vestibulocochlear* (CN VIII) contains a vestibular branch and a cochlear branch. The vestibular branch receives sensory impulses from the vestibular apparatus of the inner ear (responsible for equilibrium or balance) and forwards those impulses to the cerebellum and other areas to help maintain balance. The *cochlear branch* of this nerve receives sensory impulses from the cochlea of the inner ear (responsible for sound sensitivity) and forwards those impulses to the cochlear nuclear complex in the CNS.

   After leaving the cochlear nuclear complex, most fibers then decussate and move to the superior olivary complex, which in turn sends the fibers to the medial geniculate body in the thalamus. The thalamus then sends the fibers to Heschl's gyrus (primary hearing center) in the temporal lobe of the cortex.

   Unilateral damage that completely destroys the cochlea, auditory nerve, or cochlear nuclei will typically result in total deafness in that ear. Unilateral damage in the ascending auditory pathways and in the auditory cortex can result in impaired hearing but not total deafness because of bilateral auditory pathways. Hearing acuity problems can indirectly affect the speaker's loudness modulation, articulation, and prosody.

Unilateral or bilateral damage in Heschl's gyrus can result in auditory agnosia, which is a perceptual problem where the individual has difficulty recognizing and identifying sounds in the environment, including speech. Auditory agnosia is not due to hearing loss (hearing acuity is normal), nor aphasia (reading comprehension and oral and written expression are normal).

4. *Glossopharyngeal* (CN IX) receives sensory impulses from the posterior one third of the tongue (taste and sensation) and from the pharynx, and sends motor impulses to the pharynx for dilation, contributing to the elevation and closure of the pharynx and larynx during the act of swallowing. CN IX works along with CN X, which has the predominant control over laryngeal and pharyngeal sensory and motor function. Therefore, information concerning the effect on the speech mechanism is indicated under CN X.

5. *Vagus* (CN X) receives sensory impulses from the larynx, pharynx, soft palate, and thoracic and abdominal viscera, and sends motor impulses to the larynx, pharynx, soft palate, and visceral organs. Unilateral damage to the motor function can affect phonation (reduced loudness, short phrases, breathiness, reduced pitch range, hoarseness, diplophonia), resonance (mild hypernasality, nasal emission), and prosody (short phrases). Bilateral damage can affect phonation (short phrases, reduced loudness, breathiness, aphonia, inhalatory stridor, hoarseness, reduced pitch range), resonance (moderate to severe hypernasality, nasal emission), articulation (weak pressure consonants), and prosody (short phrases, slow rate).

6. *Spinal accessory* (CN XI) contains a spinal and cranial root. The *spinal portion* sends motor impulses to the neck and the shoulder. Unilateral or bilateral damage to the motor function can cause neck turning and shoulder elevation problems, which may indirectly affect respiration, phonation, and resonance. The *cranial portion* sends motor impulses to

the soft palate, pharynx, and larynx. CN XI works along with CN X, which has the predominant control over palatal, pharyngeal, and laryngeal motor function. Therefore, information concerning the effect on the speech mechanism is indicated under CN X.

7. *Hypoglossal* (CN XII) receives sensory and taste impulses from the tongue, and sends motor impulses to the tongue. Unilateral damage to the motor function can affect articulation (mild). Bilateral damage can affect articulation (mild to severe) and prosody (slow rate).

The 12 cranial nerves, their general function, and if damaged, their effects on the respiration, phonation, resonance, articulation, and prosody components of speech production are listed in Table 2.1. An age-old jingle to help remember the cranial nerves is "On old Olympus' towering tops, a Finn and German viewed some hops." The first letter of each word represents the first letter of each name of the cranial nerves.

The Neurosensory System

The neurosensory system is found in all the major levels of the human nervous system. Of vital importance for speech and hearing are the sensory pathways of general somatic functioning, the cranial nerves, vision and hearing, and the control circuits.

The General Somatic Pathways
The general somatic (pain, touch, temperature, and proprioception) sensory pathways dealing with the limbs and the trunk employ the spinal cord and spinal nerves. The somatic sensory pathways involved with the head and speech mechanism employ the cranial nerves (except for the process of respiration, which employs the spinal nerves). The sensory impulse from the periphery (e.g., skin of the arm or leg) is mediated and passed to the spinal nerves through the dorsal (posterior) portion of the cell body. From there, the sensory impulse moves through spinothalamic tracts to the thalamus, then through thalamocortical tracts to the internal capsule, and then onto the somatosensory area of the parietal lobe (postcentral gyrus or "sensory strip" area). Sensory

Table 2.1. The 12 Cranial Nerves and if Damaged, Their Effect on Speech Production

Cranial nerve	Function	Effect on speech production
I Olfactory	s: smell	—
	m: —	—
II Optic	s: vision	—
	m: —	—
III Oculomotor	s: —	—
	m: eye movement	—
IV Trochlear	s: —	—
	m: eye movement	—
V Trigeminal	s: jaw, lips, face, tongue	indirect—articulation
	m: jaw	articulation, prosody
VI Abducens	s: —	—
	m: eye movement	—
VII Facial	s: tongue, soft palate, nasopharynx	—
	m: face, lips, stapedius (middle ear)	articulation, prosody, facial expression
VIII Vestibulocochlear	s: vestibular—balance	—
	s: cochlear—hearing	indirect—loudness, modulation, articulation, prosody
	m: —	—
IX Glossopharyngeal	s: tongue, pharynx	—
	m: pharynx[a], larynx[a]	phonation, resonance
X Vagus	s: larynx, pharynx, soft palate, thoracic and abdominal viscera	—
	m: larynx, pharynx, soft palate	phonation, resonance, articulation, prosody
XI Spinal accessory	s: —	—
	m: spinal–neck, shoulder	indirect—respiration, phonation, resonance
	m: cranial—soft palate[a], pharynx[a], larynx[a]	phonation, resonance
XII Hypoglossal	s: tongue	—
	m: tongue	articulation, prosody

Note: s = sensory, m = motor.
[a] along with cranial nerve X.

information about proprioception is needed so that adjustments and compensations can take place when necessary (e.g., speaking immediately after dental work, talking with food in your mouth, talking after biting your tongue or cheek, etc.).

The Cranial Nerves

Some cranial nerves have only motor functions, some have only sensory functions, and some have a mixture of both functions. For the cranial nerves that are utilized for sensation, the sensory impulse from the periphery (e.g., tongue or lips) is mediated and passed to nerve cells located in the brain stem. From there, the sensory impulse is sent to the thalamus, then through thalamocortical tracts to the internal capsule, and then on to the somatosensory area of the parietal lobe (postcentral gyrus or "sensory strip" area).

The Vision and Hearing Pathways

The neurosensory system also contains special pathways used for vision and hearing. *The visual system,* under the mediation of the optic nerve (CN II), starts with the eye's absorbing light from an image, then sends the image through to the pupil. The image is then inverted and reversed as it travels into the lens. The lens focuses and projects the light onto the retina, which is a formation of nerve cells lining the inside of the eyeball. The retina sends the visual impulse to the optic nerve (this can be seen with an ophthalmoscope), which then sends it to the optic chiasma (a junction of the right and left optic nerves). At the optic chiasma, many of the fibers decussate and then move on to the lateral geniculate body of the thalamus, which then sends the fibers through the internal capsule. From there, the visual impulse is sent to the primary center for vision and the visual association areas of the occipital lobe. (Lesions of the optic nerve and the primary visual cortex can result in blindness. Lesions in the visual association cortex can result in visual perceptual problems [visual agnosia], and play a role in reading comprehension deficit [alexia].)

The neurosensory pathway used for hearing has already been noted in the section dealing with cranial nerves (under CN VIII). It is apparent that auditory and visual information is vital for the production of speech and language. The auditory system is crucial, and the visual system is quite important, in the acquisition of speech and language. The auditory system helps maintain these faculties throughout life.

The Control Circuits

The neural information that the basal ganglia and cerebellar control circuits give to the direct and indirect activation systems for their functioning, rely on the hoards of constant and instantaneous sensory information received from the periphery (e.g., proprioception, etc.).

The Autonomic Nervous System

The autonomic nervous system (ANS), which controls involuntary activity of the body, consists of a *sympathetic* and a *parasympathetic division*. The ANS is self-regulating and is present throughout the CNS and the PNS.

The sympathetic division is responsible for such activities as speeding up the heart rate, constricting the peripheral blood vessels, elevating blood pressure, raising the eyelids, redistributing blood, dilating the pupils, and decreasing contractions of the intestines. This division makes internal adjustments and alerts the body to cope with stress and crises (e.g., dilates the pupils of the eyes to allow more light to enter for better sight, distributes blood from the intestines to the skeletal muscles for strength, etc.).

The parasympathetic division is responsible for such activities as slowing down the heart rate, increasing contractions of the intestines, increasing salivation, and increasing secretions of the glands in the gastrointestines. This division is responsible for reducing internal activity and calming down the body (e.g., for digestion and bowel movement, sexual activity, etc.).

The ANS works along with the endocrine system (glands and other structures that release internal secretions called hormones) to maintain homeostasis (stability of the body's internal environment). All activity to maintain homeostasis is regulated by the hypothalamus in the CNS.

The ANS has an indirect effect upon speech and language, such as the nervousness (blushing, blanching, heart-pounding, sweating, dry mouth, or jittery stomach) that one may feel before, during, or after certain speaking situations (e.g., speaking before an audience, a marriage proposal, play acting in a speaking role, social conversation during a blind date, etc.).

CHAPTER 3

Aphasia

receptive
expressive
reading
writing

Definition

Aphasia can be defined as a multi-modality language disturbance (of the person's regular language of communication) due to brain damage. The language modalities involved are auditory comprehension, reading comprehension, oral expression, and written expression. Typically, the language components that are disturbed are the phonologic (sound system), the morphologic and syntactic (grammar), and the semantic (meaning).

The language component most preserved in aphasia is the pragmatic (social use). The wife of a severely impaired aphasia patient who was wheelchair bound once told this author that their grandchildren didn't think anything was wrong with Grandpa. At first glance, the grandchildren noticed the wheelchair and that Grandpa wasn't talking very much. In a split second, Grandpa beckoned the kids with his left hand, his facial expressions, and his general warmth. In no time, the kids were on his lap, and he was hugging and kissing and communicating with them as he usually did.

Aphasia is not caused by a motor problem affecting the person's ability to speak (e.g., paralysis of the lips), by a sensory problem affecting the ability to hear (e.g., hearing loss), or by a thought disorder affecting the ability to speak or listen (e.g., dementia). To be diagnosed as having aphasia, the person's language disturbance has to stand out in relation to the other problems. For instance, the patient with schizophrenia may have language symptoms in common with those of aphasia (see, for example, DiSimoni, Darley, & Aronson, 1977; and Halpern & McCartin-Clark, 1984). However, this patient is not identified as having aphasia because of the other apparent behavioral, thought, social, and communicative problems caused by schizophrenia.

Symptoms

Auditory Comprehension Deficit

Difficulty in the comprehension of spoken language is generally known as *auditory comprehension deficit*. The deficit is linguistic in nature and not due to perceptual (see Gandour, Holasuit Petty, & Dardarananda, 1988) or attentional (see Wiegersma, Post, Veldhuijsen, & DeVries, 1988) factors. The neuronal array for attention and perception is located in both hemispheres, with a greater representation in the right hemisphere.

If brain damage disturbs the neuronal array in a particular hemisphere, it will cause attentional and perceptual problems (neglect) in the field opposite to the involved hemisphere. Neglect problems are far greater after right rather than left hemisphere damage. Because most cases of aphasia are caused by left hemisphere damage, the chance of neglect is not great. However, some measure of neglect (Benson & Ardila, 1996) and/or attention allocation deficits (King & Hux, 1996; Murray, Holland, & Beeson, 1997, 1998; Tseng, McNeil, & Molenkovic, et al., 1993) may exist with some aphasic patients, to further compound the problem.

The individual with auditory comprehension deficit may have difficulty in understanding the following:

1. abstract words as opposed to concrete words (e.g., *The Big Apple* vs. *apple*)
2. longer words as opposed to shorter words
3. infrequently used words compared with frequently used words (e.g., *domicile* vs. *house*)

4. closely associated words (e.g., *banana* and *apple*)

5. word forms involving tense, pluralization, prefixes, suffixes, possessives, comparatives, and grammatical class

6. sentences that are long or grammatically complex (word order) or include several ideas

Brookshire (1974) has noted that some patients have a "slow rise time" where they miss the beginning of a sentence; some have a "noise buildup" where they miss the end of a sentence; some have an "information capacity deficit" where they cannot receive and process at the same time; some have a "retention deficit" where an increase in sentence length brings a decrease in performance; and some have "intermittent auditory imperception" where the patient's understanding of auditory input fluctuates.

The patient can have a reduced auditory retention span and a general slowness of comprehension.

Some factors that aid the patient with auditory comprehension deficit are as follows:

1. Pauses and imposed delays in the right spots will help the patient.

2. Stressed words are easier to comprehend, or as Kimelman (1991) noted, the words prior to the stressed word may be the important factor.

3. Vocabulary related to work, family, functional use, and recreation is easier.

4. The speaker's facial expressions, tone of voice, and use of gestures all aid the patient's comprehension. The use of a conversational tone in the form of a question will be better understood than a direct command (e.g., "Can I use your phone?" instead of "Point to the phone," or "What time is it?" instead of "Point to your watch").

5. Tompkins (1991a) has noted that aphasic patients retain knowledge of emotional meanings, and Reuterskiold (1991) found that aphasic subjects had better auditory comprehension on emotional words than on non-emotional words.

Schulte and Brandt (1989) have reviewed some non-linguistic factors that play a role in auditory comprehension deficit. They are (a) fatigue—the more tired the patient, the poorer the response; (b) scheduling—earlier in the day is better; (c) medication—side effects come into play; (d) illness—the healthier patient does better; (e) hearing loss and words that sound alike (e.g., *neck* and *leg*, *hair* and *ear*)—these can interfere with comprehension; and (f) emotional status and psychological factors—negativity and self-isolation can interfere with comprehension.

Typically, incidence of the syndrome called clinical depression is not high in aphasia (Damecour & Caplan, 1991). However, it is not uncommon for the patient to feel depressed under the combined burdens of a communication problem, a physical problem, and loss of status as breadwinner and/or homemaker (Benson & Ardila, 1996; J. Sarno, 1991; Swindell & Hammons, 1991).

Reading Comprehension Deficit

Alexia refers to an acquired impairment in reading comprehension due to brain damage. Many of the same disturbances that apply to auditory comprehension deficit can be observed in alexia, except that here the difficulty is in reading comprehension. Instead of confusing closely associated words that he or she hears (e.g., *banana* and *apple*), as in auditory comprehension deficit, the aphasic patient will confuse closely associated words that are in printed or written form.

The person's ability to read out loud is not reading comprehension. Reading out loud is going from one modality (visual) to another (speaking), with or without comprehension. For example, this author can read aloud a word, sentence, or paragraph in Spanish or German, with all the proper pronunciations and rhythms of the language; in some cases he will understand what is being read and in other cases he will not.

Benson (1979) and Benson and Ardila (1996) have described three types of alexia that are based upon the neuroanatomical site of lesion. One type called *parietal-temporal alexia* (alexia with agraphia) is associated with the fluent aphasias. The chief characteristics are the almost total loss of reading comprehension and written expression. A second type called *frontal alexia* is associated with the nonfluent aphasias. The chief characteristic is the ability to understand single words more easily than sentences. A third type called *occipital alexia* is not associated with other language problems. The major characteristic is the inability to comprehend through reading, while other language modalities are normal. Written expression is preserved, but the patient can't understand through reading what was just written correctly.

Oral Expression Deficit

Difficulty in the formulation of spoken language is called an *oral expression deficit*. The problem is most likely influenced by the same factors cited under auditory comprehension deficit, and manifests itself as the following:

1. a reduced vocabulary with infrequent words mostly gone

2. jargon, which can be unintelligible words that usually follow the phonological rules of our language (e.g., "freach") or intelligible words that bear no relationship to the stimulus

If consistent sound combinations occur that do not follow our phonemic rules, another language may be in the background of the patient. If one listens closely to jargon, one may detect whether some amount of auditory or reading comprehension is taking place. For example, when one patient was asked, "Where is your wife?" he responded with "she" in the middle of a good deal of jargon. Another, when asked, "How's the weather?" responded with jargon and "outside." Another, when asked if he was going outside, responded with jargon and "car" and "walking." Another, when asked if he would be eating soon, responded with jargon and "lunch."

3. reduced fluency (nonfluent) or excessive fluency (fluent), determined by the number of words spoken

4. circumlocutions, which can be empty speech (e.g., "The thing that's on the thing with the thing there"), a description of the use or function of the item to be named (e.g., "You carry it" or "It has handles" for *bag*), or using a word that is correct semantically and syntactically but is not in common usage (e.g., in response to "We sleep in a _____," one patient said, "tent" and another said, "building"; in response to "There is someone at the _____," a patient replied, "window")

5. neologisms, which are made up of new words that are understandable (e.g., "skymobile" for *airplane,* "windglass" for *window,* "chead" for *chin,* "inkpencil" for *pen*)

6. a semantic error or a verbal paraphasia, which represent confusion with closely associated words

The confusion can occur with words in the same category (e.g., "chair" for *table*), through description of use (e.g., "it sleep" for *bed*), with opposites (e.g., "no" for *yes*), through visual spatial contiguity (saying the name of an object or picture that is visually adjacent to the intended stimulus, e.g., there is a picture of a train passing through fields, with a cow in sight, and the patient says, "cow" for *train*), or through visual perception confusion (e.g., "fan" for *windmill*).

7. articulation errors

The misarticulation can be a substitution, omission, distortion, or addition of a sound. A substitution error is the production of a different standard sound in our language for the target (correct) sound (e.g., "<u>th</u>ing" for <u>s</u>ing). An omission error is leaving out the target sound completely (e.g., "ing" for <u>s</u>ing). A distortion error is producing a nonstandard sound in our language for the target sound (e.g., a lateral emission /s/ for <u>s</u>ing). An addition error is the production of an extra sound to the target sound (e.g., "<u>suh</u>ing" for <u>s</u>ing).

The articulation error can be at the *phonetic level,* where the sound as part of the word has been retrieved but there is a mechanical problem in producing it. This type of error typically can be found in patients with Broca's aphasia, apraxia of speech, dysarthria, or any combination of those disorders. The articulation error can be at the *phonemic* level, where the sound as part of the word is still in the process of being retrieved. This type of error, also called a literal or phonemic paraphasia, typically can be found in patients with conduction or Wernicke's aphasia (for further elaboration, see the rest of this chapter and Chapters 7 and 8). Finally, there are aphasic patients who produce few or no phonetic or phonemic articulation errors (see Darley, 1982; Halpern, Keith, & Darley, 1976).

8. grammatical errors

Grammar represents the form and structure of language and is composed of the phonologic, morphologic, and syntactic aspects of language. The phonologic aspect has been noted previously under articulation errors. *Morphology* is the system that governs the structure of words and the construction of word forms. *Syntax* is the system that governs the combination of words to form sentences, and the relationship among the elements within a sentence in order to convey meaning. Errors at the morphologic level can involve confusion with tense, pluralization, prefixes, suffixes, possessives, comparatives, and grammatical class. Errors at the syntactic level can involve confusion with word order in producing phrases and sentences.

In the language of aphasia, the words *agrammatism* and *syntactic error* have been used interchangeably to describe morphologic (word) and syntactic (sentence) errors, and the word *paragrammatism* has been used to describe syntactic errors. Following are descriptions and examples of agrammatism and paragrammatism at the sentence level.

Agrammatism is a nonfluent output that is rich in substantive words (e.g., verbs, nouns, adjectives) but sparse in function words (e.g., prepositions, pronouns, articles). Although sentences are short and constructed in a primitive manner, they frequently provide a good deal of information. A nonfluent output containing agrammatisms is also described as telegraphic or condensed speech (e.g., "Water in mouth" for *I am thirsty and would like a drink of water*).

Paragrammatism is a fluent output lacking substantive words and overusing function words. The sentences are long and without defining limits, contain verbal paraphasias and neologisms, show facile articulation, and tend toward logorrhea (pressure to speak). The sentences are lacking in semantic content and often provide little information. (One aphasic patient, when asked to *point* to the tape recorder, *spoke* without being asked to do so, and without a pause: "I've tried to all I had on my own but it doesn't make it I tried to make it but it doesn't work right why I have the recording but it was very very good but the whole part of the radio itself I've tried to do it myself I can even show it to you I haven't but what I want to say about it that is why I tried to do it by myself but I could stay and pay I would like to do it just one more minute that I would try some place to have it done." The patient was probably trying to say that his own tape recorder or radio or stereo set was in need of repair, and that he tried unsuccessfully to fix it and would now have to send it out to be repaired.)

9. word finding difficulty

This is present in all types of aphasia as well as in other neurogenic language disorders. Because word finding difficulty is so prevalent in neurogenically caused language disorders, it might be unreliable as a diagnostic indicator of a specific condition.

10. perseveration, which is the repetition of a response that is no longer appropriate

Perseveration can occur on the level of sound (soap—schair), syllable (baby—baynana), prefix (unhappy—unhat), suffix (wonderful—

childrenful), word (boy—boy), phrase (a lovely person—a lovely person), sentence (I can't say it—I can't say it), or incomplete sentence (The boy is going to the store—The boy is going bread).

11. automatic speech, which can be best described as verbal stereotypes

Typically, automatic speech is language that is overlearned, such as counting, reciting the days of the week, saying the alphabet, jingles, parts of songs, parts of prayers, curse words, etc. It's a sort of sublanguage that can appear at any time. When words are taken out of their automatic mold and put into a more formulative framework, this can cause problems for the patient (the patient is able to correctly rattle off 1, 2, 3, 4, 5, 6, 7, 8, 9, 10, but has difficulty when asked what comes after the number 3).

12. failure to respond at all, or the use of only a single word (e.g., "no no no") or part of a sentence (e.g., "I know it but I can't, I know it but I can't" or "You know it and I know it, You know it and I know it") in response to most stimuli

Many times, the response will take on the prosodic changes that reflect the mood of the patient. The patient who responded with "You know it and I know it" said it in the manner of Humphrey Bogart, James Cagney, or Clint Eastwood in their best tough-guy roles.

13. oral responses that do not fit into any of the other categories mentioned (spelling a word out loud when asked to name it or making the sound of an object when asked to name it, e.g., "vooooom" for *car* or *airplane*, or "mmmmm" for *motor*).

Written Expression Deficit

An acquired impairment in the formulation of written language due to brain damage is called *written expression deficit* or *agraphia*. Many of the problems and influencing factors cited in the other symptom categories would apply here. For example, if shown a picture of a pen, the patient responds by writing closely associated words such as *paper, ink,* or *pencil* (semantic error). The patient may write *pens* for *pen* (grammatical error), keep writing the same word over and over again inappropriately (perseveration), and so on.

It doesn't matter what sort of handwriting the patient has. The letters can be wiggly, out of line, or written in a slow, groping manner; if the language is correct, it is not agraphia. On the other hand, the letters and words can be written perfectly in a fluent and easy manner; if the language is incorrect, it is agraphia.

Benson (1979) has described two types of aphasic agraphia (see Benson & Ardila, 1996, for additional types of aphasic agraphia) that are based upon the neuroanatomical site of lesion. One type is called *dominant frontal (anterior) agraphia* and is often associated with the nonfluent aphasias and hemiplegia. Output is limited to single, substantive words with spelling errors, and if sentences are required, many short grammatical words are omitted. The mechanics of writing are large and messy.

A second type is called *dominant parietal-temporal (posterior) agraphia* and is often associated with the fluent aphasias. Output contains many spelling errors and verbal paragraphia (semantic), and if sentences are required, many patients will offer wordy, empty sentences. The mechanics of writing are normal or nearly so, and usually these patients will have no hemiplegia.

Classification

Through the years, aphasic patients have been classified in many ways. It is beyond the realm of this book to go into all of the classification systems and the controversies surrounding them (see Benson & Ardila, 1996). Several of the more popular ones are noted here. Wernicke (1874) suggested a motor and sensory division. The *motor classification* involved a lesion in the anterior cortex and included motor speech activities, whereas the *sensory classification* involved a lesion in the posterior cortex and included auditory reception activities.

Weisenburg and McBride (1935) gave us *expressive, receptive,* and *mixed expressive and receptive* classifications. With this classification system, expressive aphasia was linked with anterior lesions, and receptive aphasia was linked with posterior lesions. Because almost all aphasia patients show deficits in the four language modalities (auditory comprehension, reading comprehension, oral expression, and written expression), the Wernicke and Weisenburg and McBride classifications appeared too vague and thus lost their momentum as tools for diagnosis. However, their classification systems led to a division based on *anterior* or *posterior* site of lesion; most aphasiologists associate an anterior lesion with the motor and expressive classification, and a posterior lesion with the sensory and receptive classification.

Currently, there are three popular ways to classify aphasic patients. One method is assessing patients as having a mild, moderate, or severe impairment. In this approach, the symptoms appearing in the various modalities are described and given a ranking of impairment within each modality and/or across all the modalities.

Aphasia can also be classified into *nonfluent aphasia,* usually caused by damage to anterior portions of the language-dominant side of the brain, and *fluent aphasia,* usually caused by damage to posterior portions of the language-dominant side of the brain. Authors such as Benson (1979), Benson & Ardila (1996), Davis (1993), and Goodglass and Kaplan (1983) have reviewed both types as follows. Nonfluent aphasia is characterized by

1. decreased output (50 words or less per minute, and often fewer than 10 words per minute);

2. increased effort in producing speech;

3. defective articulation (because of the last two characteristics, prosody may be abnormal);

4. decreased phrase length (fewer than 4 words, and often only single words per phrase);

5. primitive syntax but a lot of information conveyed;

6. fewer paraphasias of the phonemic (literal), verbal (semantic), neologistic, and jargon types;

7. awareness of impairment and, as a result, frustration.

Fluent aphasia is characterized by

1. increased output (mostly within the normal range of 100–150 words per minute, and sometimes as high as 200 words per minute);

2. effortless production of speech;

3. relatively normal articulation (because of the previous two characteristics, prosody may be normal);

4. normal phrase length (about 5 or more words per phrase);

5. long sentences without defining limits, a lot of meaningless, empty talk characterized by a lack of substantive words, and a tendency toward logarrhea (a pressure to speak);

6. many paraphasias of the phonemic (literal), verbal (semantic), neologistic, and jargon types;

7. frequent lack of awareness of the impairment and, as a result, no frustration over the condition.

A third way of categorizing aphasia is by site of lesion. The *perisylvian* area (Benson, 1979; Benson & Ardila, 1996; H. Damasio, 1991) is located around the lateral fissure in the dominant hemisphere and contains the major language areas used for comprehension and expression (Figure 3.1). The aphasias caused by lesions in the perisylvian area would include Broca's, Wernicke's, and conduction. The *borderzone* area (Benson, 1979; H. Damasio, 1991) or *extrasylvian* area (Benson & Ardila,

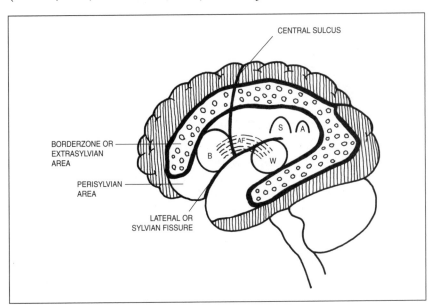

Figure 3.1. Lateral view of the left hemisphere (dominant) showing the location of the borderzone or extrasylvian area and the perisylvian area where B is Broca's area, W is Wernicke's area, AF is the arcuate fasciculus, S is the supramarginal gyrus, and A is the angular gyrus.

1996) of the dominant hemisphere is located outside the perisylvian area, in the vascular borderzone between the territory of the middle cerebral artery and the territory of the anterior or posterior cerebral artery (Figure 3.1). The aphasias caused by lesions in the borderzone area would include transcortical motor aphasia, transcortical sensory aphasia, and mixed transcortical aphasia (isolation of the speech area). The aphasias caused by a nonlocalizing lesion would include anomic and global.

Nonfluent Aphasia Syndromes

The nonfluent aphasias typically include Broca's aphasia, transcortical motor aphasia, global aphasia, and mixed transcortical aphasia or isolation syndrome.

Broca's Aphasia

Broca's aphasia is characterized by a sparse output of words and sentences, misarticulations, and agrammatisms. Speech is laborious, filled with many pauses, and is telegraphic. Auditory and reading comprehension are better than oral expression, and written expression tends to mirror oral expression. Repetition of words, phrases, and sentences is poor. The right side of the body is often paralyzed, and patients are aware of their difficulties, which can lead to frustration or catastrophic reaction (extreme emotional behavior such as complete withdrawal, prolonged crying, and intense hostility when the patient is unable to cope with demands made upon him or her).

Typically, the lesion (H. Damasio, 1991) is in the posterior portion of the frontal lobe of the dominant hemisphere. It is in the perisylvian zone and may involve not only Broca's area but also premotor and motor regions immediately behind and above (Figure 3.1). In addition, the lesion may involve the underlying white matter and basal ganglia, as well as the insula, which is in the paralimbic area and may be seen by pulling apart the two borders of the lateral fissure (or the fissure of Sylvius).

Transcortical Motor Aphasia

Transcortical motor aphasia is similar to Broca's aphasia, with the exception that these patients have the ability to repeat words, phrases, and sentences. It is a relatively rare syndrome. Generally, the lesion (H. Damasio, 1991) is in the frontal lobe of the dominant hemisphere, is anterior or superior to Broca's area, and lies within the borderzone region (Figure 3.1). It is either deep in the left frontal substance or in the cortex.

Global Aphasia

Global aphasia consists of a severe impairment in auditory and reading comprehension, and oral and written expression. Patients try to communicate but often can produce only verbal stereotypes and automatic speech. Repetition of words, phrases, and sentences is defective. Nonlanguage perceptual and problem-solving abilities may be impaired (nonlanguage abilities are mostly intact in the other types of aphasia). Mostly, the lesion (H. Damasio, 1991) involves a widespread area of the perisylvian zone of the dominant hemisphere, affecting all areas whose damage correlates with the aphasias (Figure 3.1).

Mixed Transcortical Aphasia

Mixed transcortical aphasia or isolation syndrome is similar to global aphasia, except that these patients can repeat and show echolalia of words, phrases, and sentences. It is a relatively rare syndrome. Mostly, the lesion (Benson & Ardila, 1996) involves a widespread area of the anterior and posterior borderzone regions of the dominant hemisphere (Figure 3.1).

Fluent Aphasia Syndromes

The fluent aphasias typically include Wernicke's aphasia, transcortical sensory aphasia, conduction aphasia, and anomic aphasia.

Wernicke's Aphasia

Wernicke's aphasia is characterized by fluent, verbal paraphasic, and generally well-articulated speech. Jargon, neologisms, and empty speech are common features. Auditory and reading comprehension and written expression are impaired. Repetition of words, phrases, and sentences is poor. Patients show few or no other neurologic signs and are often unaware of their errors, which leads to less incidence of frustration. On the other hand, some of these patients can become suspicious or even paranoid about their circumstances.

Generally, the lesion (H. Damasio, 1991) is in the posterior portion of the temporal lobe of the dominant hemisphere. It is in the perisylvian zone involving Wernicke's (left superior temporal gyrus) and surrounding areas (Figure 3.1).

Transcortical Sensory Aphasia

Transcortical sensory aphasia is similar to Wernicke's aphasia, except that these patients have the ability to repeat and show echolalia of words, phrases, and sentences. It is a relatively rare syndrome.

Mostly, the lesion (H. Damasio, 1991) is in the posterior portion of the temporal or parietal lobes; in the middle temporal gyrus or occasionally in the angular gyrus, in the white matter underlying these cortices, or a combination of both. The lesion is in the borderzone area in the dominant hemisphere (Figure 3.1).

Conduction Aphasia

Conduction aphasia consists of fluent, verbal, and phonemic paraphasic speech, although usually less severe than that in Wernicke's aphasia. Auditory and reading comprehension are relatively good, whereas written expression is defective. Repetition of words, phrases, and sentences is disproportionately severely impaired in relation to the level of fluency in spontaneous speech, and the near normal level of auditory comprehension. Other motor signs may be present, and because of the patient's awareness of errors, his or her speech can be filled with unsuccessful attempts at self-correction.

Typically, the lesion (H. Damasio, 1991) can be in the arcuate fasciculus (the fibers that connect Wernicke's area with Broca's area) or deep in the supramarginal gyrus. The lesion can also be in a subsylvian involvement of Wernicke's area, in the primary auditory cortex, or to a variable degree, the insula and its subcortical white matter. The lesion is in the perisylvian area in the dominant hemisphere (Figure 3.1).

Anomic Aphasia

Anomic aphasia is characterized by fluent, well-articulated, mildly paraphasic, grammatically intact, and somewhat empty speech. The outstanding symptom is a naming or word-finding problem that can affect any of the modalities. Generally, if other symptoms appear, they do so mildly in the various modalities. These patients have no difficulty with repetition of words, phrases, and sentences. They know when they make errors, and because of unsuccessful attempts at self-correction, they often become frustrated. As mentioned previously, word-finding difficulty is probably the most common symptom found in aphasia and other neurogenically caused language disorders. Many times, word-finding difficulty is the only residual symptom as the patient gets better.

Generally, the site of lesion (H. Damasio, 1991) is variable, but damage to the left anterior temporal cortices is an essential element.

Aphasia in Bilingual or Multilingual Individuals

In their review, Benson and Ardila (1996) looked at whether bilingual or polyglot (multilingual) aphasic patients show equal impairment in the different languages, or better recovery in just one of them. Those who observe that one language recovers better than the others cite such factors as the language learned early in life, the language most consistently used at the onset of aphasia, and the language milieu during recovery. Benson and Ardila have concluded that no set pattern exists for the recovery of language in the bilingual or polyglot patient.

Additional Sources

For a further review of the various symptoms and classifications of aphasia, and site of lesion, the reader is referred to Benson (1979), Benson & Ardila (1996), Brookshire (1997), Code (1989), A. Damasio (1991), H. Damasio (1991), Davis (1993), Goodglass and Kaplan (1983), Hegde (1998), Love and Webb (1996), and Swindell, Holland, and Reinmuth (1998).

Etiology

As was stated in the definition, aphasia is caused by brain damage, most likely in the cortical language areas of the left hemisphere. In some cases, aphasia can occur because of lesions in subcortical areas, mostly in the thalamus or basal ganglia. In some cases, a lesion in the right hemisphere of a right-handed person will cause a crossed aphasia.

A major cause of aphasia in middle and old age is the *cerebrovascular accident* (CVA). Cerebrovascular accidents consist of *thromboses, embolisms, aneurysms, hemorrhages,* and *ischemias*. A cerebral thrombosis is an occlusion of an artery to the brain by a clot. A cerebral embolus is a clot formed elsewhere that finally lodges in the brain. An aneurysm is a swelling or ballooning of a cranial artery. A cerebral hemorrhage is the rupture of a blood vessel with subsequent bleeding into the brain. Ischemia refers to deficient circulation in the brain. All cerebrovascular accidents have one thing in common: they deprive the brain of oxygen and circulation, thus causing brain damage.

Trauma to the brain is another major cause of aphasia. Gunshot wounds, automobile accidents, and falls are the most likely causes of physical trauma to the brain. Brain tumors, both malignant and nonmalignant, are associated with aphasia. Quite often, the extirpation of a brain tumor will cause aphasia. This author remembers one young man in his early 20s who suffered symptoms of brain damage (spasms, blackouts, etc., but no aphasia). A diagnostic workup determined that a brain tumor was present in his left frontal lobe. Although the tumor was benign, the surgery left him with aphasia and a right-sided paralysis. Abscesses, infectious diseases, and degenerative disease of the brain can also result in aphasia.

Progressive Aphasia

Occasionally, an ongoing cerebral atrophy in a language area of the brain can result in progressive language deterioration. If the person's nonverbal memory and intellect remain intact, the language deterioration is known as a *progressive aphasia*.

Duffy and Peterson (1992) reported on 54 cases of progressive aphasia. They found the main features of this condition to be as follows:

1. Age of onset ranged from 40 to 75, with a mean of 59.3 years.
2. More males were affected than females, by a ratio of 2 to 1.
3. The duration of the isolated language symptoms ranged from 1–15 years, with a mean of 5.3 years.
4. Autopsy findings for 14 cases revealed Pick's disease in 4, Creutzfeldt-Jakob disease in 3, Alzheimer's disease in 3, focal spongiform degeneration in 2, and nonspecific cellular degeneration in 2. The

variation of neuropathology does not support the notion that a specific disease causes the isolated language decline. It must be noted that Pick's, Alzheimer's, and Creutzfeldt-Jakob diseases are known causes of dementia.

5. Computed tomography CT-scans were reported for 47 cases. Of these scans, 13 were normal, 5 indicated diffuse abnormality, 10 showed greater left than right abnormality, and 19 indicated left hemisphere abnormality only.

6. Most of the cases had fluent, anomic, or Wernicke's-like aphasia. Twelve cases had a nonfluent or Broca's-like aphasia and sometimes an accompanying apraxia of speech.

As a result of their review, Duffy and Peterson concluded that progressive aphasia has been reported frequently enough to be considered a separate and distinct clinical–behavioral entity.

Additional Sources

Reviews of etiology of aphasia can be found in Benson (1979), Benson & Ardila (1996), Brookshire (1997), Brown and Perecman (1986), Davis (1993), and Mlcoch and Metter (1994).

Diagnosis

Procedures for diagnosing aphasia can involve (a) establishing background information, (b) giving a neurologic evaluation, (c) employing four-modality tests, (d) employing functional language tests, (e) employing single-modality tests, and (f) evaluating connected speech.

Establishing Background Information

Establishing background information about the neurogenic patient with a communication disorder can involve obtaining *basic, medical,* and *related area information* through questioning the patient and/or the caretaker, and through access to medical and other reports. Procedures for establishing background information are applicable to the other language and motor speech disorders discussed in this book.

Basic information can include the patient's name, age, educational level, occupation, marital and family status, previous speech, language, and cognitive problems, family history of speech, language, and cognitive problems, native language, and communicating language.

Medical information can include the onset and course of the disorder, diagnosis of the disorder, past illnesses, any injuries, general physical condition, past cerebrovascular disorders, previous central or peripheral nervous system damage, disorientation, confusion, paralysis, seizures, loss of consciousness, chronic conditions, and instrumentation findings (CT scan, etc.).

Related area information can include visual deficits, hearing deficits, pre-onset personality, post-onset personality, mood changes, memory functioning, swallowing, drooling, medications which may have affected speech, language, and cognition, substance abuse (alcohol, etc.), and the patient's awareness and perception of the problem.

The Neurologic Evaluation

The neurologic evaluation includes those procedures used in determining the type of pathology and the location of the brain lesion. These neurodiagnostic procedures are applicable to the other language and motor speech disorders discussed in this book.

Benson and Ardila (1996) have reviewed the localization techniques used in determining the neuroanatomical site of brain damage in cases of aphasia. The localization techniques include neuropathology, neurosurgery, posttrauma skull defects, the neurologic examination, and brain-imaging studies.

Neuropathology relies upon direct postmortem anatomical observation of patients who had suffered language impairment. *Neurosurgery* correlates the site of surgical incision and the subsequent aphasia; and prior to surgery the focal stimulation of brain areas (with the patient awake and responding to questions) and its correlation to the elicited language symptoms. *Posttrauma skull defects* correlates the site of skull damage and the aphasic symptoms.

The neurologic examination involves a visual sensory examination that checks for visual-field defects, a motor examination that checks for paralysis, a sensory examination that checks for pain and/or temperature loss, and a motor praxis examination that checks for apraxia. The defects in these areas are then correlated to the neural system responsible for their functioning.

Brain-imaging studies include *isotope brain scans, cerebral blood flow and metabolism studies, computed tomography* (CT), and *magnetic resonance imaging* (MRI). An isotope brain scan involves an injection of an isotope followed by counts of radioactivity over brain areas. Cerebral blood flow and metabolism studies involve the use of positron isotopes, as in positron emission tomography (PET) studies, which provide relatively precise neuroanatomical delineation based on variations in glucose metabolism. Dynamic isotope studies reveal brain areas with increased blood flow or alterations of metabolic rate when the subject performs certain activities. Single-photon emission-computed tomography (SPECT) uses relatively stable isotope products to demonstrate cerebral blood flow and, to a lesser degree, perfusion of metabolites.

Computed tomography (CT) relies on the penetration of X-ray beams processed through computerized mathematics, which provides a tomographic (pictures of body section) image of the brain without physical invasion of the body. Magnetic resonance imaging (MRI) uses a powerful magnetic field to alter electrical fields in the brain, which can then be monitored electronically to produce computerized images (slices) of brain tissues. MRI does not use X-ray and does not introduce radioactive material into the patient's body.

In addition to the above, Brookshire (1997) describes the use of *X-rays* (for observing the skull and/or spine), *cerebral angiography* (for observing the veins and arteries of the brain and brain stem), *myelography* (for observing the spinal cord and spinal nerves), *B-mode carotid imaging* (for observing extracranial blood vessels with ultrasound), *electroencephalograms (EEG)* (for obtaining a graphic record of the electrical activity of the cerebral cortex), *electromyography* (for recording the electrical activities of muscles), *nerve conduction studies* (for measuring stimulation and response points along the nerve fiber), *lumbar punctures* (for analyzing a sample of cerebrospinal fluid), and *biopsies* (for analyzing samples of tissue).

Four-Modality Tests

Most of the tests used for aphasia evaluate all four modalities. Each modality is tested individually, with stimulus items generally ranging from simple to more complex. For example, auditory comprehension might be tested by the examiner's saying single words, multiple words, sentences, and paragraphs to the patient (e.g., "Point to the window") and having him or her respond by pointing, nodding, or gesturing in response to the auditory stimuli. Reading comprehension might be tested by the examiner's presenting printed words, sentences, and paragraphs to the patient (e.g., *Do cows fly?*) and having him or her respond by pointing to, circling, or underlining the printed words *yes* or *no*, or by nodding or gesturing.

Oral expression might be tested by having the patient produce sub-language items such as serial speech (e.g., reciting the alphabet or days of the week) and repeating words after the examiner, and language items such as sentence completion (e.g., "We sleep in a __."), naming pictures or objects, defining words and sentences, and talking spontaneously about everyday activities. Written expression might be tested by having the patient produce sub-language items such as copying letters and words and writing words to dictation, and language items such as writing the name of an object or item shown in a picture and writing a narrative from an action picture.

Tests that evaluate the four modalities in the manner described include the following: *Acute Aphasia Screening Protocol* (AASP) (Crary, Haak, & Malinsky, 1989); *Aphasia Language Performance Scales* (ALPS) (Keenan & Brassell, 1975); *Bedside Evaluation Screening Test* (BEST) (Fitch-West & Sands, 1987); *Bilingual Aphasia Test* (BAT) (Paradis, 1987); *Boston Assessment of Severe Aphasia* (BASA) (Helm-Estabrooks, Ramsberger, Morgan, & Nicholas, 1989); *Boston Diagnostic Aphasia Examination* (BDAE) (Goodglass & Kaplan, 1983); *Examining for Aphasia* (Eisenson, 1954); *Language Modalities Test for Aphasia* (LMTA) (Wepman & Jones, 1961); *Minnesota Test for Differential Diagnosis of Aphasia* (MTDDA) (Schuell, 1972); *Multilingual Aphasia Examination* (MAE) (Benton & Hamsher, 1978); *Neurosensory Center Comprehensive Examination for Aphasia* (NCCEA) (Spreen & Benton, 1969); *Porch Index of Communicative Ability* (PICA) (Porch, 1981); *Sklar Aphasia Scale* (SAS) (Sklar, 1973); and *Western Aphasia Battery* (WAB) (Kertesz, 1982). Of the above tests, the AASP omits evaluating reading comprehension, and the BEST omits evaluating written expression.

Currently, the most popular tests are the BDAE, MTDDA, PICA, and WAB. The BDAE and the WAB are the only tests that place patients in the classic aphasia categories of Broca's, transcortical motor, global, mixed transcortical, Wernicke's, transcortical sensory, conduction, and anomic. The other tests place patients in the mild, moderate, and severe impairment categories or have specialized categories (e.g., the MTDDA contains the categories of simple aphasia, aphasia with visual involvement, aphasia with sensorimotor involvement, aphasia with scattered findings compatible with generalized brain damage, and irreversible aphasic syndrome. Two minor syndromes are aphasia with partial auditory imperception and aphasia with persisting dysarthria).

Functional Language Tests

Some tests evaluate functional language through the various modalities. Many times these tests are used as adjuncts to the more traditional tests used for aphasia. They include the following: *ASHA Functional Assessment of Communication Skills for Adults* (ASHA FACS) (American Speech-Language-Hearing Association, 1994); *Assessment Protocol of Pragmatic-Linguistic Skills* (APPLS) (Gerber & Gurland, 1989); *Communicative Effectiveness Index* (CETI) (Lomas et al., 1989); *Communicative Abilities in Daily Living* (CADL) (Holland, 1980); and *Functional Communication Profile* (FCP) (Sarno, 1969).

Items in these tests elicit language related to everyday activities (greetings, shopping, family matters, etc.), and the tests are administered in a relatively informal manner. The authors of these tests feel that because of the emphasis on functional language or social-communicative interaction and the informal setting, the psychological barriers of tension and anxiety that accompany formal test taking would be ameliorated.

Single-Modality Tests

Other tests evaluate the patient's language abilities through only one modality. Usually, these tests evaluate in depth and are quite sensitive, thus enabling the detection of even the mildest language impairment. These tests are used mostly as adjuncts to the more traditional ones and include the following: *Auditory Comprehension Test for Sentences* (ACTS) (Shewan, 1980); *Boston Naming Test* (BNT) (Kaplan, Goodglass, & Weintraub, 1983); *Reading Comprehension Battery for Aphasia* (RCBA) (LaPointe & Horner, 1980); *The Reporters Test* (DeRenzi & Ferrari, 1978), which evaluates oral expression; *The Token Test* (DeRenzi & Vignolo, 1962), which evaluates auditory comprehension; *Revised Token Test* (RTT) (McNeil & Prescot, 1978); and *Word Fluency Measure* (Borkowski, Benton, & Spreen, 1967), which evaluates oral expression.

Evaluating Connected Speech

As an adjunct to the aphasia tests mentioned previously, several studies have looked at the connected speech of aphasic adults as a means for evaluation.

Nicholas and Brookshire (1995b) noted that various measures have been used to compare the connected speech of aphasic adults to that of non–brain damaged adults, and to evaluate changes in connected speech over time. Such measures range from those used to assess adherence to standard language rules and patterns of use to those used to evaluate the informativeness and efficiency of connected speech.

Measures of adherence to standard language rules and patterns of use include counts of syntactic errors (Shewan, 1988; Wagenaar, Snow, & Prins, 1975); ratio of clauses to terminal units (Hunt, 1965); and type-token ratio, mean length of utterance, and number and types of cohesive ties (Halliday & Hasan, 1976). Measures of communicative informativeness and efficiency include content units per minute (Yorkston & Beukelman, 1980a); percent of words that are correct information units (Nicholas & Brookshire, 1993); presence, completeness, and accuracy of main concept production (Nicholas & Brookshire, 1995a, b); and subjective ratings of coherence (Ulatowska, Freedman-Stern, Doyel, & Macaluso-Haynes, 1983).

Recently, the *Discourse Comprehension Test* (Brookshire & Nicholas, 1997) was designed to assess listening and reading comprehension, and retention of stated and implied main ideas and details from narrative discourse. The authors maintain that the test is appropriate for adults with aphasia, right hemisphere brain damage, or traumatic brain injury. Main idea questions test central information that is repeated or elaborated on by other information in the story. Detail questions test peripheral information that is mentioned only once and not elaborated on by other information in the story. Stated questions test information that appears in a story in essentially the same form in which it is subsequently tested. Implied questions test information that is not directly stated but has to be inferred from other information in the story; answering these questions requires the listener to form bridging assumptions and draw inferences.

Nicholas and Brookshire (1995a), using an earlier version of the *Discourse Comprehension Test*, found that the performance of groups of patients with brain damage (20 patients had left hemisphere brain damage and aphasia, 20 had right hemisphere brain damage, and 20 had traumatic brain injury) was qualitatively similar to that of the group with no brain damage (40 subjects), but quantitatively inferior. The performance of the groups with brain damage was qualitatively and quantitatively similar. The performance of all groups was strongly affected by the salience of information in the stories. All 100 subjects responded correctly to main idea questions more often than to detail questions. The effect of directness was less strong than that of salience, but all groups produced more correct responses when questions assessed stated information than when they assessed implied information. The effect of directness was greater for detail questions than for main idea questions.

Additional Sources

Finally, for all of the tests mentioned, if a complete evaluation is not made during the initial diagnostic session, additional sessions may be required to ascertain the full picture of the patient's abilities.

Reviews of testing procedures for aphasia and other adult neurogenic communication disorders can be found in Benson and Ardila (1996), Brookshire (1997), Chapey (1994), Davis (1993), Golper and Cherney (1999), Haynes, Pindzola, and Emerick (1992), Peterson and Marquardt (1994), and Spreen and Risser (1991).

Therapy

There are three basic goals of therapy that are applicable to all the communication disorders described in this book.

The first goal is to inform the patient and the caretaker(s) about the nature and consequences of the disorder. This is done to help alleviate any misconceptions about the condition and to provide the proper counseling and psychological support for the patient and the caretaker(s). Information about spontaneous recovery, prognosis, stages of the disorder, and reactions of the patient and/or family may be included in this goal.

The second goal is to provide the appropriate treatment approaches and techniques. This is done to teach the patient how to compensate and use various strategies in his or her efforts to communicate in a functional manner. Information about the efficacy of therapy may be included in this goal.

The third goal is to encourage the patient and the caretaker(s) to continue the rehabilitative process outside of the clinical setting. This would involve practice and environmental changes at home or at the care facility to achieve the carry over or generalization of what occurs in the clinical setting. Information about family and spousal attitudes, and general and specialized home or facility treatment by caretakers may be included in this goal.

The first goal of therapy is to inform the patient and the caretaker(s) about the nature and consequences of the disorder.

After a language evaluation is completed, usually the speech–language pathologist, and occasionally another professional, will relate the findings to the patient and/or caretaker. It makes life a little easier for the patient and caretaker if the one explaining the evaluation can say where needed, "You have a condition called aphasia, and all aphasia means is a language disturbance. Your thinking abilities should be close to normal. Aphasia is very common after strokes (or trauma or tumor). You have no motor problems of the lips or tongue (or you have a motor problem, dysarthria or apraxia of speech, and that is why your articulation is disturbed). Your brain is healing every second and with that can come some restoration of function. Of course, everybody is not the same. Some will heal faster than others."

The above sounds so obvious, but this author has dealt with a number of patients and caretakers who were still completely in the dark about the condition even after seeing the appropriate professionals. One aphasic patient came to the rehabilitation center for his therapy on a bus. Using his aphasic language along with gestures, he explained that people on the bus and elsewhere thought that he was either drunk (forming his hand like a cup and making a drinking motion) or crazy (moving his index finger in a circle near his right temple). Uninformed or poorly-informed patients and caretakers may feel the same way about the condition called aphasia.

Spontaneous Recovery

Before getting into the specifics of therapy, there are several factors that influence the language intervention process. One factor is the concept of spontaneous recovery, which is the body healing itself without any therapy. Spontaneous recovery is most likely due to a reduction of edema or swelling in the damaged hemisphere, a return to normal blood flow or circulation in the undamaged hemisphere, and collateral or compensatory blood circulation in the damaged hemisphere.

The greatest amount of spontaneous recovery takes place within the first 2 months postonset of the brain lesion. More spontaneous recovery will take place from the 3rd through the 6th month postonset, but to a lesser extent than in the first 2 months. More recovery will take place from the 7th through the 12th months, but this will not be as much as in the first 6 months. Reviews of spontaneous recovery can be found in Benson (1979), Benson and Ardila (1996), Davis (1993), Kertesz, Lau, and Polk (1993), and M. Sarno (1991).

Prognosis

Prognosis is another feature in language rehabilitation. Before deciding who would make a good candidate for therapy or providing information to patients and their families about the prospects for improvement, the clinician could gain insight into these processes through a number of prognostic indicators. These indicators might also predict improvement through spontaneous recovery.

Although the prognostic factors cited are gleaned from the literature in aphasia, many of these indicators might apply to patients with other communicative disorders. The following prognostic indicators have been outlined by Benson & Ardila (1996), Brookshire (1983), Brookshire (1997), Darley (1982), Davis (1993), and M. Sarno (1991).

1. The younger the patient, the better the prognosis.

2. The sooner the patient enters therapy after the onset of aphasia, the better the prognosis.

3. The less extensive the neurological damage, the better the prognosis.

4. Borderzone and subcortical lesions offer a better prognosis than perisylvian lesions.

5. Broca's, transcortical motor, conduction, and anomic aphasia offer a better prognosis than the other types of aphasia.

6. Hemorrhage as a cause of cerebrovascular accident seems to offer a better prognosis than ischemia.

7. If the aphasic patient has the will to improve and accept his or her limitations, the prognosis is better.

8. If the family of the aphasic patient has the proper attitude and provides encouragement to the patient, the prognosis is better.

9. The milder the language impairment at the initial evaluation, the better the prognosis.

10. If the patient receives a longer and more intense period of speech and language therapy, the prognosis is better.

11. The better the physical condition with no sensory defects, the better the prognosis.

Darley (1982) cited several studies indicating that when dysarthria accompanies aphasia, the prognosis for recovery in aphasia is poorer. However, other studies he cited differed about prognosis when apraxia of speech or oral apraxia accompanies aphasia. Although there are always exceptions, these prognostic factors might provide insight and guidelines for therapy and help in guidance and counseling procedures for the family.

Patients' Reaction to Illness

Aphasic patients may react to their illness with depression, anxiety, denial, guilt at being sick, anger, counterproductive coping, fear, frustration, and embarrassment. This author remembers one 75-year-old, wheelchair-confined aphasic patient, whose nephew built a wooden ramp with handrails leading from the house to the backyard. With the ramp providing easy access, the patient still refused to sit in his own backyard because he was embarrassed to have the neighbors see him sitting in a wheelchair.

Patients may also have emotional lability and catastrophic reactions (Damecour & Caplan, 1991; Sapir & Aronson, 1990; Swindell & Hammons, 1991). These reactions can interfere with the whole rehabilitative process, especially language therapy. As Damecour and Caplan (1991) noted in their study of aphasic patients, depression was not correlated with lesion site or size of lesion, and there was no difference in the degree of depression between Broca's and Wernicke's subjects.

The second goal of therapy is to provide the appropriate treatment approaches and techniques.

Efficacy of Aphasia Therapy

There are two types of research design used in studies to determine the efficacy of aphasia therapy. There are *group studies,* which measure the effects of aphasia therapy (in its various forms) as opposed to no therapy or deferred therapy, or the effects of therapy administered by speech–language pathologists as opposed to trained volunteers. The findings of each study are generalized to the greater population. Group study research includes that of Basso, Capitani, and Vignolo (1979), Butfield and Zangwill (1946), David, Enderby, and Bainton (1982), Deal and Deal (1978), Elman and Bernstein-Ellis (1999), Hartman and Landau (1987), Lincoln et al. (1984), Marshall et al. (1989), Meikle et al. (1979), Poeck, Huber, and Willmes (1989), Sarno, Silverman, and Sands (1970), Shewan and Kertesz (1984), Vignolo (1964), Wertz et al. (1981), and Wertz et al. (1986).

There are also *single-subject experimental studies,* which measure the effectiveness of specific forms of aphasia therapy administered to an individual patient over a period of time and checked at designated intervals. The findings of each study are applicable only to the individual subject, not to the general population. See, for example, the single-subject studies of Boyle and Coelho (1995), Kearns (1985), McNeil, Small, Masterson, and Fossett (1995), and Thompson, Shapiro, and Roberts (1993).

By almost all accounts (whether the studies are of group or single-subject design), it appears that language therapy for the aphasic patient is beneficial for language recovery. As Robey (1994) noted in his analysis of 21 efficacy of treatment studies, there is a clear superiority in the performance of aphasic patients who receive treatment from a speech–language pathologist.

In a follow-up meta-analysis of 55 reports of aphasia treatment outcomes, Robey (1998) found the following:

1. Results for treated patients are superior to those for untreated patients in all stages of recovery. Results are greatest when therapy is begun in the acute stage of recovery (during or before the 3rd month post-onset of the neuropathology).

2. Therapy length of 2 hours or more per week brings more gains than does therapy of shorter durations.

3. Of specifically named therapies, the Schuell-Wepman-Darley Multimodality (SWDM) or "stimulation approach" was reported in a relatively large number of primary studies.

4. Large gains are achieved by severely aphasic patients when they are treated by a speech–language pathologist.

5. There are too few investigations that examine the differential effects of therapies for the different types of aphasia.

Recently, Elman and Bernstein-Ellis (1999) found that adults with chronic aphasia receiving group communication treatment (5 hours per week) had significantly higher scores on linguistic and communicative measures than adults with chronic aphasia not receiving treatment. In addition, significant increases were revealed after 2 months of treatment and after 4 months of treatment.

Holland, Fromm, DeRuyter, and Stein (1996) have noted several representative treatment techniques that appear to be effective with aphasic patients. These treatment approaches and techniques include the following (described later in this chapter): traditional modality specific stimulus-response treatment (also known as the "stimulation approach"), language oriented therapy (LOT), group therapy, functional communication therapy, PACE therapy, programmed instruction approaches, melodic intonation therapy, and visual action therapy. Holland et al. (1996) wrote, "Talented aphasia clinicians sample from among available approaches for those that augment their patient's strengths and compensate for deficits. . . . Matching aphasic patients to the most effective clinical technique for management is an area ripe for further investigation" (p. s33).

In conclusion, Brookshire (1994) has stated

> The work is not yet over, for several issues remain—issues which are likely to escalate in importance as resources allocated to health care diminish and as accountability becomes more and more important. Aphasiologists need to demonstrate that specific treatment approaches work for specific communicative disabilities. Although single-case studies seem a natural vehicle for this work, it may be that group studies will be needed to convince consumers (patients, families, physicians, and funding agencies) that the approaches are appropriate and effective for some meaningful segment of the aphasic population. (p. 12)

The literature on the efficacy of aphasia therapy has been reviewed by Brookshire (1994), Davis (1993), Elman and Bernstein-Ellis (1999), Holland et al. (1996), Robey (1994, 1998), and Wertz (1992).

Stimulation Approach

One of the major approaches to aphasia therapy is the stimulation approach and its variations. As Darley (1972) has stated,

> In the stimulation approach the goal of therapy is to stimulate the patient to produce cortical integration necessary for language, not to educate or re-educate him and not to convey specific new learning or new vocabulary. . . . That stimulus must be adequate and it must get into the brain. It involves repetitive sensory stimulation, each stimulus eliciting a response. (pp. 12–13)

For specifics and a further elaboration of this method of aphasia therapy, the reader is referred to Brookshire (1997), Darley (1982), Davis (1993), Duffy (1994), Rosenbeck, LaPointe, and Wertz (1989), Santo Pietro and Goldfarb (1995), Schuell, Jenkins, and Jimenez-Pabon (1964), and Wepman (1951).

Duffy (1994) reviewed and analyzed the stimulation approaches to aphasia therapy. He noted that the use of intensive controlled auditory stimulation is supported by the following: (a) sensory stimulation affects brain activity; (b) repeated sensory stimuli are essential for the organization, storage, and retrieval of language patterns in the brain; (c) the auditory system is of prime importance for language acquisition and for processing information and feedback in ongoing functional language; (d) nearly all aphasic patients have auditory deficits, and recovery in this modality will help the other modalities; (e) because of its crucial link to language, gains made through the auditory modality will extend to all other input and output language channels.

General Principles of the Stimulation Approach

Duffy (1994) further reviewed the general principles of the stimulation approach. They are presented here along with additional references: (a) intensive auditory stimulation should be used along with the other modalities; (b) the stimulus must be adequate and get into the brain; (c) repetitive sensory stimulation should be used; Hough, Pierce, and Cannito (1989) and Tompkins (1991b) found that redundancy of stimulation will help comprehension in aphasia; (d) each stimulus should elicit a response; (e) responses should be elicited and not forced; (f) a maximum number of responses should be elicited; a large number of adequate responses indicates a large number of adequate stimuli; (g) feedback about accuracy of response should be provided when such feedback appears beneficial; (h) work should proceed systematically and intensively; (i) sessions should begin with relatively easy, familiar tasks and proceed to more difficult tasks after the patient experiences success; (j) the examiner should use abundant and varied materials and present them in the proper manner. Bracy and Drummond (1993) found that the use of pictograms (comic strips) was better than a single picture for eliciting word retrieval in fluent and nonfluent aphasic subjects; (k) new materials and procedures should be extensions of familiar materials and procedures.

Structure of Stimulation

The structure of stimulation listed below follows the Duffy (1994) outline. Many of the research summaries surrounding each factor can be found in Brookshire (1997), Darley (1982), Duffy (1994), and Rosenbek et al. (1989), along with additional references.

Auditory perceptual clarity (volume and noise). Reducing noise or working in quiet facilitates language performance. Increasing volume is not useful except in specific cases.

Nonlinguistic visual-perceptual clarity (dimensionality, size, color, content, ambiguity, operativity). Operativity is described as a stimulus that can involve other senses. For example, a picture of a rock will be easier for the patient to name than a picture of a cloud. A rock can be seen and touched, whereas a cloud can only be seen. Operativity may be another term for concreteness. The clinician should be clear, realistic, and redundant. The most potent visual stimuli are characterized by three dimensions, color, lack of ambiguity, operativity, and redundant physical properties.

Quite often, for a confrontation naming task, this author uses very large (8 ½" × 11") and very clear black and white pictures from a popular rehabilitation kit. However, one picture is that of an open box of matches, with the matches lined up in the rectangular box. Many patients have perceived a piano from the shape of the box, with the lineup of matches as a line of piano keys.

Towne and Banick (1989) studied the naming performances of nonfluent and fluent aphasic adults. They found no significant differences in naming ability when subjects were presented with black and white or colored versions of pictures.

Linguistic visual-perceptual clarity (size and form). Large print seems better; the clinician should be aware of idiosyncratic preferences.

Method of delivery of auditory stimulation. Auditory stimulation that is direct, with live voice, binaural, and in the free field, is best.

Discriminability (semantic, auditory, visual). The best approach is to select stimuli that offer few response alternatives. In the semantic area, words that are closely associated in meaning (e.g., *knife* and *fork*) should be avoided when the patient is given a number of responses from which to choose. Similarly, closely related choices should be avoided when presenting words auditorily (e.g., *goat* and *coat*) and visually (e.g., *car* and *oar*). The clinician should particularly avoid stimuli that contain two or three of the factors mentioned above (e.g., *ear* and *hair*; *neck* and *leg*), where they can be confused semantically and auditorily.

Stimulus repetition. Repetition of stimuli after the incorrect response appears to increase adequate responses.

Rate and pause. The clinician should speak slowly with a slow overall rate. He or she should pause at appropriate intervals to help auditory retention, and reduce rate of phoneme production by prolonging words (see Goldfarb & Halpern, 1981; Schulte & Brandt, 1989).

Length (a factor in all modalities). Through the visual modality, short words, sentences, and paragraphs are better; through the auditory modality, short phrases, sentences, and paragraphs are better. Length may not be a factor at the word level. Redundancy can overcome the limitations of length. For example, Halpern (1965a, b) and Silver and Halpern (1992) found that regardless of modality, long words were more difficult for aphasic patients than were short words.

Combined sensory modalities. The best method is combined auditory and visual stimulation. This helps the single modalities and is a good starting point. Using the tactile modality also helps. The multimodality stimulus provides redundancy and additional cues for the patient. The patient shouldn't be overloaded with too much multimodality stimulation. It can cause distraction and exceed the capacity of the patient.

Beukelman, Yorkston, and Waugh (1980) found that aphasic patients are more successful when given combined verbal and pantomimed instructions than when given these instructions separately. Hough (1993) treated a Wernicke's aphasia patient who had jargon using a program concentrating on visual and written stimuli instead of auditory comprehension activities. After 2 months, the patient improved in naming and general conversation, including a reduction of the jargon.

Cues, prompts, and prestimulation. These are techniques to facilitate word finding in oral and written expression, or in auditory and reading comprehension (some examples of this are given in this chapter). Freed and Marshall (1995), Freed, Marshall, and Nippold (1995), and Lowell, Beeson, and Holland (1995) elaborate further on the use of cues, prompts, and prestimulations in aphasia therapy.

Frequency and meaningfulness. Frequency refers to how often a word is used in the English language. Meaningfulness refers to language that contains personal relevance and emotion, and whose content conforms to the expected order of things (e.g., *Dog bites man* rather than *Man bites dog*). The higher the frequency of occurrence in the language (see Halpern, 1965b; Silver & Halpern, 1992) and the more meaningful the word stimuli, the greater the chance of a correct response.

Abstractness. Concrete words represent items that are closely related to the senses (e.g., *apple*, one can see, touch, smell, and hear the biting crunch of an apple), whereas abstract words represent concepts that are distant from the senses (e.g., *justice, mercy*). Abstractness can be overcome by frequency of occurrence and redundancy. Redundant (semantically supporting) words in a sentence may facilitate comprehension regardless of abstraction level or even length (e.g., "Point to the furry cat" would be easier for the patient than "Point to the cat" in an array of pictures placed in front of the patient).

Part of speech. Verbs, adjectives, and nouns may be easier than conjunctions, articles, and prepositions. Among verbs, adjectives, and nouns, nouns would likely be easiest if frequency is controlled (see Halpern, 1965b).

Grammatical considerations. There is a hierarchy of grammatical difficulty that affects all the aphasias. In any modality, the harder the grammar, the more difficulty the aphasic patient has. For example, present-tense sentences (e.g., *The boy catches the ball*) are easier to comprehend than past-tense sentences (e.g., *The boy caught the ball*) or future-tense sentences (e.g., *The boy will catch the ball*). Sentences that use the agent-action-object order (e.g., *The mother hugs the baby*) are easier than sentences that do not use this order (e.g., *The policeman was kicked by the robber*). Sentences that are simplified syntactically by expansion (e.g., *The woman was tall and the man was short*) are easier than grammatically compact sentences (e.g., *The woman was taller than the man*).

Other, morphologic or syntactic features indicate that comprehension or expression of the affirmative is easier than the negative, singular easier than plurals, and plurals easier than possessives (e.g., *horses* vs. *horse's*).

These are just a few examples of how grammatical complexity can affect the aphasia patient.

Stress. This factor appears to be tied to word order and saliency. Kimelman (1991) found that stressed target words alone within a paragraph did not bring better auditory comprehension in aphasic listeners. The author postulated that better auditory comprehension was probably due to the prosodic cues that preceded the stressed target words.

Saliency is characterized by stress and phonological prominence and by informational and personal significance. Not only will aphasic patients do better with auditory comprehension when stress is employed, but they will also be more successful when asked to repeat sentences that contain salient features (e.g., "Sink or swim, he said" is easier for the patient to repeat than "He said, sink or swim"). Many patients need a salient word at the beginning of the utterance in order to initiate speech.

Order of difficulty. The clinician should begin with familiar, easy tasks, then proceed to less familiar and more difficult ones, and end with tasks that result in a great deal of success.

Psychological and physical factors. Patients do better when not suffering from tension or fatigue. Tompkins, Marshall, and Phillips (1980) found that mornings are better than afternoons for scheduling therapy.

Pattern of auditory deficit. As mentioned previously under symptoms, Brookshire (1974) noted that in comprehending sentences, patients can show any of the following: slow rise time (miss initial portions); noise buildup (miss final portions); retention deficit (length causes problems); information capacity deficit (too many ideas in sentences); intermittent auditory imperception (understanding of auditory input fluctuates randomly).

Concerning response characteristics, short responses are easier for the patient. The speech–language pathologist should choose the easiest modality for the patient and see whether the patient responds best in unison with the stimulus, immediately following the stimulus, or after a delay. The response characteristics of accuracy, recognition, and attempts at self-correction should all be considered. Marshall and Tompkins (1981) offered a review of the self-cueing and self-correction behaviors of aphasic patients. The clinician should give patients continuous feedback on their responses.

Specific Examples of the Stimulation Approach

Following are some suggestions for therapy for deficits in the four language modalities. These suggestions derive from the general literature in aphasia and from this author's own experience. Within each modality, the tasks gradually move from easy to more difficult items. Each task listed is only one example of what could develop into any number of other tasks.

Therapy for auditory comprehension deficit (ACD). In the following tasks, the clinician provides the auditory stimulus. The patient responds in the different manners described. In those tasks requiring the use of pictures, the number of pictures can range anywhere from one to six.

Starting with auditory comprehension of single words (ACD 1.B), the clinician can place a single picture (e.g., of a key) or a single object (e.g., the key itself) in front of the patient. The clinician can identify the picture or the object by pointing to it and naming it several times. After that, the clinician says "key," "Point to the key," or "Show me the key," and beckons for the patient to respond by pointing to the picture or the object.

When convinced that the patient understands, the clinician can introduce another stimulus word (e.g., *spoon*) and work with only that word in the manner described above. The next step would be putting the two pictures or the two objects (e.g., key and spoon) side by side. The clinician proceeds by saying one of the two stimulus words and having the patient indicate the correct picture or item.

If the patient is correct according to whatever criterion the clinician uses (e.g., correct 90% or better over a number of tries), then the clinician can introduce additional stimulus words in the same manner. If the patient is not correct at the level of two stimulus words, the clinician should return to a single stimulus word and introduce some of the other modalities to reinforce the auditory modality (e.g., showing the printed stimulus word, having the patient write it, and/or having the patient say it in addition to hearing it from the clinician).

Many of these procedures described as a starting point for auditory comprehension can be converted into a starting point for reading comprehension (e.g., instead of saying the stimulus word to the patient, the clinician can match the printed stimulus word to the picture or the object, as in RCD 3.A, and proceed as outlined for auditory comprehension).

ACD   1. A. Commands involving the body (e.g., "Look up, look down, stand up, sit down, close your eyes, open your eyes, turn around, stick out your tongue, smile, take off your glasses, put on your glasses," etc.).
     B. Point to picture matching single word stimulus.
     C. Point to own body parts or clothing matching single word stimulus (e.g., *nose, shirt*).

          D. Point to items in room matching single word stimulus (e.g., *lamp, door*).

ACD 2. A. Point to picture showing antonym to single word stimulus (e.g., *up–down*).

          B. Point to picture showing semantic association for single word stimulus (e.g., *table–chair*).

          C. Point to picture corresponding to single word nouns (e.g., *pen, carpet*).

          D. Point to picture corresponding to single word adjectives (e.g., *tall, fat*).

          E. Point to picture corresponding to single word verbs (e.g., *smiling, walking*).

          F. Point to picture corresponding to single word prepositions (e.g., *on, in*).

ACD 3. A. Follow commands to open, close, show, raise, hold, hum, shake, tap, rub, straighten, look, give, blink, put, scratch, move, touch, pucker, turn, nod, stick out, pick, make, or gesture (using self with and without objects).

ACD 4. A. Point to a printed letter or number.

          B. Point to a printed word.

          C. Point to a picture or object in order to complete a sentence (e.g., "Please pass the salt and ___").

          D. Point to a picture or object whose name is spelled (e.g., "T-A-B-L-E").

ACD 5. A. Point to a picture or object described by function (e.g., "Point to the item used for drinking").

          B. Point to a picture or object grouped by location (e.g., "What do you find in a living room?").

ACD 6. A. Point to two or three nouns (e.g., *lamp, chair, window*).

          B. Point to two or three verbs (e.g., *walking, reading, sleeping*).

          C. Point to two or three items described by function (e.g., *drinking, cutting, writing*).

          D. Point to two or three items grouped by location (e.g., "What do you find in a bedroom, living room, and kitchen?").

ACD   7. A. Point to three or four items (e.g., pictures, self, environment).
           B. Point to item described by varying number of descriptors (e.g., "Point to the small, red square").
           C. Point to item best described by a sentence (e.g., "Point to the picture of people relaxing." There will be a picture of people relaxing on a beach among other very different pictures).
           D. Follow two object location commands (e.g., "Put the pencil in front of the book").
           E. Follow two verb commands (e.g., "Point to the book, pick up the pencil").
           F. Follow two verb time commands (e.g., "Before touching the comb, pick up the cup").

(The following section requires yes/no responses from the patient.)

ACD   8. A. Questions about pictures (e.g., "Is the girl walking?").
           B. Questions involving general information (e.g., "Was Washington the 16th President?").
           C. Questions involving auditory retention span (e.g., "Are peaches, apples, pears, chickens, and bananas all fruits?").
           D. Questions involving semantic discrimination (e.g., "Do you play tennis with a bat?").
           E. Questions involving phoneme discrimination (e.g., "Do men wear shirts and pies to work?").
           F. Questions involving specific and general information from sentences and from short and long paragraphs.

(The following section requires oral or written expression, or reading comprehension responses from the patient.)

ACD   9. A. Listen to short or long paragraphs or stories and answer questions about them.
           B. Listen to short or long paragraphs or stories and retell them.

Therapy for reading comprehension deficit (RCD). In the following tasks, the clinician provides the visual stimulus in varying conditions. The patient responds to the visual stimulus in the different manners described. Many of the items suggested for auditory comprehension deficit can be converted into therapy tasks for reading comprehension deficit.

RCD   1.   A.   Match identical pictures.
             B.   Match geometric forms (e.g., □ ▽ ○ ● with ○ □ ● ▽)
             C.   Match printed letters, words, phrases, and sentences.
             D.   Match similar pictures in the same category (e.g., palm, fir, and maple trees).

(The following section requires some of the patient's auditory comprehension and oral expression abilities.)

RCD   2.   A.   Identify named letters to printed choices.
             B.   Identify named words to printed choices.
             C.   Identify multiple named words to printed choices.
             D.   Name individual printed letters.
             E.   Read in unison with the clinician.

RCD   3.   A.   Match printed word to picture or object.
             B.   Match printed word to picture using antonyms (e.g., *up–down*).
             C.   Match printed word to picture using semantic associations (e.g., *table–chair*).
             D.   Match printed phrase to picture (e.g., *brushing hair*).

RCD   4.   A.   Read simple phrase and complete (e.g., *Cats and* [*oceans, dogs, lamps*]).
             B.   Read complex phrase and complete (e.g., *A car* ___ [*travels, auto, fires*] fast).
             C.   Arrange printed words into a phrase (e.g., *of, soup, bowl*).
             D.   Arrange printed words into categories (e.g., *animals, fruits, cities*).

RCD   5. A. Read simple sentence and complete (e.g., song lyrics, *The bells are* ___ or nursery rhymes, *Jack and Jill went up the* ___).
     B. Read complex sentence and complete (e.g., *The horse has 4* ___ [*legs, ears, tails*]).

RCD   6. A. Match printed sentence to picture (e.g., *The door is open*).
     B. Read simple sentence and give yes/no response (e.g., *Is ten less than four?*).
     C. Read complex sentence and give yes/no response (e.g., *If the water is boiling, is the water cold?*).
     D. Read sentence—choice (e.g., *A state in the U.S. is* ___ [*Spain, June, Texas*]).
     E. Read sentence—homonyms (e.g., *On his shoes, he wore rubber* ___ [*heels, heals*]).
     F. Read sentence—verbs (e.g., *Mom is* ___ [*doing, do*] *the dishes*).
     G. Read sentence—plurals (e.g., *My friend has two* ___ [*son, sons*]).
     H. Read sentence—synonyms (e.g., *Another word for big is* ___ [*large, thin, small*]).
     I. Read sentence—antonyms (e.g., *The opposite of tall is* ___ [*fat, long, short*]).
     J. Read sentence—comparative (e.g., *He is* [*tall, taller, tallest*] *than she is*).
     K. Read sentence—time (e.g., *Look at the window, after you point to the floor*).

RCD   7. Follow commands (see ACD 3. for examples).

RCD   8. A. Read a short to long paragraph and give yes/no responses.
     B. Read a short to long paragraph and give multiple choice responses.

(RCD 9 and 10 require oral or written responses from the patient.)

RCD   9. A. Read single word or sentence and define.

      B. Read sentence containing *wh* questions and respond in any manner (*What? Where? When? Why? Whose? Which?*).

      C. Read a proverb and tell what it means.

RCD 10. Read a short or long paragraph, or a story, and retell it.

Therapy for oral expression deficit (OED). In the following tasks, the clinician provides stimuli in varying conditions. The patient responds orally. Many of the items suggested for auditory and reading comprehension deficit can be converted into therapy tasks for oral expression deficit.

Some suggestions for correcting erroneous responses are given in the section titled "Specific Examples for Correcting an Incorrect Response." This section follows the section titled "Therapy for written expression deficit (WED)."

OED 1. A. Repeat after clinician, read aloud, or recite automatic language (e.g., numbers, days of week, months of year, alphabet).

      B. Sing in unison with clinician or alone (e.g., "Happy Birthday," "Three Blind Mice," etc.).

      C. Say nursery rhymes in unison with clinician, repeat after clinician, or say alone (e.g., "Jack and Jill," "Humpty Dumpty," etc.).

      D. Repeat after clinician single words, phrases, sentences.

(In OED 2 & 3, the clinician says most of the phrase or sentence and the patient completes it.)

OED 2. A. Complete phrase with familiar paired associates (e.g., "bacon and ___").

      B. Complete phrase with familiar paired antonyms (e.g., stop and ___").

      C. Complete sentence with initial phonemic cue (e.g., "You blow your n___").

      D. Complete familiar sayings (e.g., "Have a good ___").

E. Complete song lyrics (e.g., "Row, row, row your ___").

F. Complete nursery rhymes (e.g., "Jack and Jill went up the ___").

OED 3. A. Complete sentence using nouns (e.g., "We sleep in a ___").

B. Complete sentence using adjectives (e.g., "The sky is ___").

C. Complete sentence using verbs (e.g., "When hungry, you should ___").

D. Complete sentence using prepositions; clinician shows pictures or objects (e.g., "The spoon is ___ the cup").

E. Complete sentence using antonyms (e.g., "He isn't fat; he's ___").

F. Complete sentence using proverbs (e.g., "Don't put all your eggs in one ___").

OED 4. A. Name pictures, objects, or body parts. Schwartz and Halpern (1973) found that naming of body parts may be affected by the physical impairment of the aphasic patient.

B. Complete sentence using convergent stimuli (e.g., "A bee makes ___").

C. Complete sentence using divergent stimuli; clinician shows pictures or objects (e.g., "I see a ___").

D. Name through function (e.g., "Name an appliance used for cooking").

E. Name through comparison (e.g., "Name an animal that's faster than a turtle").

F. Name through categories (e.g., "Name a fruit").

G. Name through semantic association (e.g., "Name as many things as you can that are white"). Ochipa, Maher, and Raymer (1998) reported that naming through semantic association was a successful intervention strategy in anomia.

OED 5. A. Say words that start with certain letters (general, male and female names, fruits, cities, etc.).

            B. Say associated words after clinician gives word (especially useful when related to patient's special interest). Goldfarb and Halpern (1981) found that in word association tasks, aphasic subjects had more difficulty in providing paradigmatic responses (words belonging to the same grammatical class, i.e., *hum* and *sing*) than syntagmatic responses (a grammatical continuation, i.e., *hum* and *tune*). Characteristics of the stimulus word that caused the most problems in evoking paradigmatic responses were high level of abstraction, short, verbs, and infrequent occurrence.

            C. Say words that rhyme, (e.g., "hot–___").

            D. Say antonyms (e.g., "up–___").

            E. Say synonyms (e.g., "car–___").

OED 6. A. Answer *wh* questions, in single words or sentences (e.g., "What barks?").

            B. Complete sentence using an adjective and noun (e.g., "Santa is wearing a ___").

            C. Formulate sentences in response to pictures.

            D. Formulate sentences in response to manipulated objects using prepositions (e.g., after placing a spoon [in, beside, in front of, behind, on, etc.] an object, the clinician asks, "Where is the spoon?").

            E. Formulate sentences in response to questions about self (e.g., age), family (e.g., names of children), general information (e.g., president of U.S.).

            F. Formulate sentences using various parts of speech (e.g., nouns, verbs).

            G. Formulate a sentence using two particular words (e.g., *find, radio*).

            H. Formulate a sentence using three particular words (e.g., *path, park, walk*).

        I. Formulate a sentence beginning or ending with selected words or phrases (e.g., "I eat," "when," "if," "she").

OED 7. A. Define words or sentences in response to auditory and/or visual stimuli.

        B. Explain the functions of items or persons (e.g., *pen, razor, tailor*).

        C. Describe what is happening in a picture.

        D. Describe the activity of the clinician as he or she moves objects about.

        E. Explain what to say in certain situations (e.g., "You are tired, so you say ___").

        F. Ask questions to find out information.

OED 8. A. Explain more than one meaning of word and then put that word in a sentence (e.g., *spring*).

        B. Explain the meaning of phrases (e.g., "blowing off steam").

        C. Explain how items are different (e.g., *pencil–crayon*).

        D. Explain how items are similar (e.g., *bus, bicycle, car*).

        E. Answer general questions (e.g., "Why do people go to school?").

        F. Explain why statements do not make sense (e.g., "Apples and carrots are fruits").

OED 9. A. Explain each step in a particular activity (e.g., "How would you make eggs for breakfast?").

        B. Describe everything possible about pictures or objects (e.g., physical properties, uses).

        C. Converse generally about selected topics (e.g., favorite TV programs, movies).

        D. Formulate summaries of short and long paragraphs (read or heard).

OED 10. A. Explain what an expression means (e.g., "The movie was so-so.").

        B. Unscramble words of a proverb and then tell what it means.

    C. Have an open-endeded conversation on unrestricted topics.

    D. Retell a radio or TV broadcast or familiar story.

    E. Take a side on a debatable question (e.g., capital punishment).

    F. Explain the ideas of well known people (e.g., Abraham Lincoln, Franklin D. Roosevelt).

    G. Explain the meaning of metaphors (e.g., "She's the apple of his eye.") and similes (e.g., "happy as a clam").

Therapy for written expression deficit (WED). In the following tasks, the clinician provides stimuli in varying conditions. The patient responds in writing. Many of the items suggested for other modalities, especially oral expression deficit, can be converted into therapy tasks for written expression deficit.

Some suggestions for correcting erroneous responses are given in the section titled "Specific Examples for Correcting an Incorrect Response." This section follows the tasks for written expression deficit. Although geared for correcting oral expression responses, many of the suggestions can be adapted for correcting written expression responses. For instance, Example 1 could easily apply to naming ability (WED 3.A). Instead of calling for an oral response, the clinician could call for a written response.

WED 1. A. Trace or copy (lines, geometric forms, numbers, letters).

      B. Trace or copy words.

      C. Write letters, numbers, words, phrases, and sentences to dictation.

WED 2. A. Fill in missing letters or words with or without associated picture stimuli (e.g., *She is writing a lette-, She is writing a ___*).

      B. Put (write) words into proper categories from choices that are mixed up (e.g., clothing, sports, fruits).

      C. Find two words embedded in one word and write them (e.g., *mailman*).

WED 3. A. Write names of pictures, body parts, or objects.
   B. Fill in the blank to make another word (e.g., *fort* ___).
   C. Write associated word for stimulus word.

WED 4. A. Complete sentences using verbs (e.g., *Children like to* ___ *in the sandbox*).
   B. Complete sentences using nouns (e.g., *On Sunday, he read the* ___).
   C. Complete sentences using adjectives (e.g., *He wore a red and* ___ *tie*).
   D. Complete sentences using prepositions (e.g., *Jack jumped* ___ *the candlestick*).
   E. Complete sentences using antonyms (e.g., *The policeman signaled stop and* ___).

WED 5. A. Complete series with words in same category (e.g., *Paris,* ___; *apple,* ___; *carrot,* ___).
   B. Write words in alphabetical order.
   C. Write several examples for each topic (e.g., items that are round, items that sail).
   D. Write words in correct order (e.g., *Quiet be, cup a coffee of*).
   E. Rewrite sentences (e.g., *That boy are going to school*).
   F. Write a sentence using a particular word.
   G. Sentence completion—divergent (e.g., *I see* ___).

WED 6. A. Write functional information (e.g., name, address, age).
   B. Write answers to questions (e.g., "What can you do with an empty bottle?").
   C. Fill out forms (e.g., bank, insurance, government).

WED 7. A. Write sentences in response to pictures or objects.
   B. Complete a story with additional sentences.
   C. Complete a crossword puzzle.

WED 8. A. Write as much as possible about a particular topic (e.g., *vacation*).

      B. Write a summary of a paragraph that clinician has narrated.

      C. Write a paragraph in response to pictures, objects, or clinician's activity.

      D. Write responses to divergent tasks (e.g., "Write three things every good citizen should do"; write the meaning of proverbs).

Specific Examples for Correcting an Incorrect Response

Following are some specific examples of how the speech–language pathologist might correct an incorrect response. If the patient fails, any one or combination of the following procedures, as reviewed by Goldfarb and Halpern (1989), might be used to correct him or her. The following procedures can also be adapted for the written expression deficit tasks suggested in WED 3. and WED 4.

Example 1

Task: Name a picture of *bread*.

1. Integral stimulation ("Watch me and listen to me"): clinician says, "bread," patient repeats.

2. Cueing: clinician shapes own articulators for "b" sound, clinician provides an eating gesture.

3. Association: clinician says, "You eat it, make toast, put butter on it," etc.

4. Completion: clinician says, "I will put butter on the___; in the bakery, I buy___").

5. Multi-modality: saying and writing *bread*, saying and seeing the printed word *bread*, saying, seeing the printed word, and writing *bread*.

6. Repetition: patient repeats the correct response (e.g., three times in a row to make sure it sticks).

7. Rhyming: clinician says, "sounds like tread, shred, head."

Example 2

Task: Provide the last word to complete a high associative open-ended sentence (or, with some modifications, turn it into a confrontational naming task).

Cues: initial phoneme, sentence completion, semantic association, and printed word.

Program: Present 25 trials, using all four cues noted above. When the patient achieves a criterion level of 80% correct responses for 25 trials over three consecutive sessions, cues will be deleted in order, first the printed word, then the initial phoneme, and finally the semantic association cue.

Examples: Although a minimum of 25 different sentences are required for each session, only 2 are used here as examples. The program is presented on four levels. Failure of the patient to achieve criterion level indicates that the speech–language pathologist should return to a previous level for a particular sentence.

> Level I. Hold a flash card with *DOOR* printed in one-inch block letters in front of the patient. About 5 seconds may be optimal. Say to the patient, "Someone is knocking at the d___." Use a similar orthographic cue for "Wash your hands with soap and w___."
>
> Level II. Present sentences as on Level I, but eliminate the flash cards.
>
> Level III. Present sentences as on Level II, but eliminate the phonemic cue.
>
> Level IV. Present open-ended sentences that do not include semantic association, such as "I don't like ___," "I see a ___," or "There is a ___."

PACE Therapy

Some forms of aphasia therapy favor an overall communication approach. One such procedure is Davis and Wilcox's (1981) PACE (Promoting Aphasics' Communicative Effectiveness). This form of therapy is based on the following four principles:

1. The speech–language pathologist and patient participate equally as senders and receivers of messages (take turns selecting a picture and conveying the message between them).

2. There is an exchange of new information between the clinician and the patient (keep pictures face down).

3. The patient has a free choice of communication modes in sending the message (use of verbal and nonverbal modalities).

4. When receiving a message from the patient, the clinician provides feedback based on whether or not the message was conveyed (a patient may be linguistically inept but communicatively superb).

The clinician can go first by picking up a picture (e.g., a man shaving) from a group of pictures that were face down. The clinician has to describe the picture verbally or through gesture. The patient has to receive this information and indicate that he understands. The patient then takes his or her turn at picking up a picture and describing it to the clinician. Pictures can show individuals who are shaving, brushing their teeth, eating, saluting, waving, etc., and can be either professionally made or come from magazines or newspapers. Davis and Wilcox (1981) advocate using PACE as an adjunct to traditional therapy because it gives the patient experience in overall communication.

Functional Communication Therapy

Another overall communication approach is Functional Communication Therapy (FCT) (Aten, 1994). The following tasks are used to elicit any manner of response (verbal, gesture) from the patient: saying name ("Your first name is ___"), greetings, ordering coffee and meals in a restaurant, address and telephone number, naming family members, occupation and hobbies, branch of service, where they grew up, make of car, favorite foods, how they like foods cooked, favorite movies, favorite TV shows, favorite vacations.

Variations of PACE and FCT can easily be adapted for patients with specific capabilities and deficits. For example, the speech–language pathologist can present a single printed word to the patient (reading comprehension) with the spoken instruction (auditory comprehension) to tell what the word means using any form of communication (oral expression, gesture, pointing). Lyon (1992) has reviewed the various forms of communication in natural settings for adult aphasic patients.

Therapy for Global Aphasia

Treatment for global aphasic patients is based on the premise that they can learn a number of skills including matching, copying, and imitation. The main justification for training patients in these sub-language areas is that it could lead to functional communication (see Collins, 1991).

For the global patient, the following unique forms of therapy are suggested:

1. The clinician should use stimuli that offer the best chance of a correct response, such as sentence completion ("The bells are ___"), automatic speech (e.g., counting, reciting the days of the week), singing, repeating after the clinician, etc. Wallace and Canter (1985) found that severely involved patients do better with personally relevant items, and Van Lancker and Klein (1990) found that global aphasia patients do better with familiar personal names.

2. Auditory comprehension of body commands appears easier than other auditory comprehension tasks. Commands that can be used are, "Stand up," "Sit down," "Turn around," "Take off your glasses," "Put on your glasses," "Put on the light," "Turn off the light," "Look up," "Look down."

3. Card games such as "21" or "Casino" might be used to elicit language or gesture. Patients can match, sequence, pick up, turn over, put, or arrange cards according to color, suit, or number.

4. Patients can visually match forms, figures, postures, and letter tiles.

5. Patients can trace, copy, and write forms, numbers, letters, and words.

6. The patient can match pantomime with a picture or imitate a gesture made by the clinician (e.g., waving, saluting).

7. Adaptations of PACE (Davis and Wilcox, 1981) and Functional Communication Therapy (FCT) (Aten, 1994), along with Visual Action Therapy (VAT) (Helm-Estabrooks, Fitzpatric, & Barresi, 1982), can be used to elicit some form of communication from the patient. VAT is

described as a nonverbal method for severe aphasic patients. With objects and line drawings of objects such as a hammer, screwdriver, cup, razor, salt shaker, etc., the patient is taught to trace, match, and demonstrate the object's use through pantomine. Although VAT is centered on a nonverbal approach, gains in auditory comprehension have been noted by Helm-Estabrooks et al. (1982).

8. Another method is visual communication therapy (Gardner, Zurif, Berry, & Baker, 1976), which is designed to teach the global patient artificial language using a system of arbitrary symbols that represent syntactic and lexical components.

One of the goals in working with global patients is to find that language breakthrough which, for example, might move the patient from a global to a Broca's category. Repeated stimulation in letter and word matching with letter tiles might lead to formulative letter spelling with tiles, or repeated auditory comprehension of body commands might lead to other forms of auditory comprehension. When there is a little opening or breakthrough, the clinician wants to "send in all the troops" with more advanced forms of therapy. Reviews of therapy for the global patient can be found in Collins (1983, 1991), Peach and Rubin (1994), and Salvatore and Thompson (1986).

Group Therapy

Kearns (1994) has reviewed the five approaches for group therapy with aphasia patients. In the first approach, the group setting acts as a vehicle for direct language treatment. Whatever is used in individual therapy is now used in the group. For example, patients may be asked to identify various objects around the room in response to auditory and reading comprehension stimuli ("Point to the chair"), or patients may be asked to name objects around the room through oral or written expression.

The second approach for group therapy involves indirect language treatment. In a loosely structured manner, activities such as general conversation, role playing, field trips, discussion of current events or other topics of interest, and general social interchange (e.g., coffee and cake servings, playing cards or checkers) are instituted.

The third approach calls for the use of sociolinguistic treatment groups. Patients engage in social functional language activities as derived from PACE, FCT, etc., types of therapy.

The fourth approach is the transition group that gears the patient for going from the clinical situation to the real-life situation. These groups meet for a limited and specific period of time prior to the patient's discharge from therapy.

The fifth approach is the maintenance group, where the patient attends stroke clubs or other groups for the disabled. These groups are very social in nature with a good deal of indirect language stimulation activities.

Marshall (1993) found that weekly attendance at group therapy that focused on functional situations was successful for mild aphasic patients. Reviews of group therapy can be found in Brookshire (1997), Darley (1982), Davis (1993), and Kearns (1994).

Programmed Instruction Therapy

Another general approach to aphasia treatment is programmed instruction. Holland (1970) has noted that programmed instruction is one example of applying learning principles to education. A program is created wherein the principles of shaping and reinforcement are used in a learning task. Shaping involves moving in small, carefully controlled steps toward closer and closer approximation of the criterion behavior. Reinforcement consists of affirmative statements as to the adequacy of a response, or merely the forward movement or progression through a program based upon a correct response.

Language-Oriented Treatment

Language-Oriented Treatment (LOT) (Shewan & Bandur, 1986) is an example of a specific treatment approach for aphasic patients that includes the principles of programmed instruction. LOT is based on the premise that in aphasia, the language system itself and access to the language system can both be disturbed. This is a view of aphasia not as a loss of language, but rather as an impairment of specific components of language (phonologic, syntactic, semantic, or any combination of these).

An example of the language system itself being impaired would be a patient who makes syntactic errors in oral expression and in auditory comprehension. An example of impairment in the access to the language system would be a patient who can write a word but cannot say it. The content of LOT is based upon a psycholinguistic approach that reflects knowledge about language, its organization, its processing, and its recovery from brain damage. The specific areas in LOT involve the following modalities: (a) auditory processing, (b) visual processing, (c) gestural and combined gestural-verbal conversation, (d) oral expression, and (e) graphic expression.

Base-Ten Programmed Stimulation Method

In a rather unique combination of the stimulation and programmed instruction approaches, LaPointe (1977) developed the Base-Ten Programmed Stimulation Method. Included in this method are the programmed operant procedures of clearly defined tasks, baseline performance measurement, and session-by-session progress plotting of the aphasia patient. This is combined with the numerous features of the stimulation approach designed to elicit many responses from aphasic patients.

With the programmed stimulation approach, speech and language tasks are composed of 10 stimulus items, which are scored and plotted during 10 therapy sessions. This method also includes compensatory-facilitative and self-cueing strategies that are useful for some aphasic patients in oral expression and auditory comprehension.

Other Therapy Approaches

Other approaches to aphasia therapy include Melodic Intonation Therapy (MIT) (Sparks & Deck, 1994), and the Voluntary Control of Involuntary Utterances (VCIU) (Helm & Barresi, 1980), both of which are described in the therapy section of Chapter 8 in this book. The Helm Elicited Language Program for Syntax Stimulation (HELPSS) (Helm-Estabrooks, 1981) is an approach designed to stimulate agrammatic or paragrammatic aphasics' access to syntactical knowledge. This program is for use with nonfluent aphasic patients and includes training of 11 sentence types with a story completion format.

A number of computer systems for use with specific aphasic problems have been reviewed by Katz and Wertz (1997); these include programs for verbal word finding, verbal sentence construction, auditory comprehension, single-word visual recognition, single-word reading comprehension, homophone recognition, written spelling, and written word finding.

In their own study, Katz and Wertz (1997) found that computerized reading treatment for chronic aphasic adults showed the following: (a) The tasks could be administered with minimal assistance from a clinician; (b) improvement on the computerized reading treatment tasks generalized to non-computer language performance; (c) improvement resulted from the language content of the software and not stimulation provided by a computer; and (d) the computerized reading treatment was efficacious.

The third goal of therapy is to encourage the patient and the caretaker(s) to continue the rehabilitative process outside of the clinical setting.

Family Attitudes

One of the prognostic variables mentioned earlier noted that if the family of the patient has the proper attitude and provides encouragement, then the prognosis is better. Most families desire the best for the aphasic patient and would do anything to make him or her communicatively normal. Because of their feelings for the patient, family members might look at the patient's language abilities unrealistically.

On a number of occasions, this author has had family members sit in during a therapy session. After watching and listening to a 30- to 45-minute session where the patient showed little or no response to the most basic auditory comprehension stimuli, the family member will say, "But he (the patient) understands everything." Or, after observing a diagnostic or therapy session that is devoted partially or fully to oral expression, the family member will say, "She is too stubborn to talk" or "She thinks it's too simple and that's why she doesn't want to talk."

Spousal Attitudes

Helmick, Watamori, and Palmer (1976) found that spouses of aphasic patients view the patients' communication as less impaired than it actually is. Zraick and Boone (1991) noted that the attitudes most frequently expressed by spouses of aphasic patients were that the aphasic spouse was demanding, temperamental, immature, worrisome, and nervous. This was not typical of the control subjects. Spouses of nonfluent aphasic patients showed most of the above attitudes, and spouses of fluent aphasic patients showed the fewest of these attitudes. Spouses of the nonfluent group viewed the patients as less independent, less compliant, and less sociable than their fluent patient counterparts. The authors postulated that this may be due in part to the nonfluent patients' absence of words and/or struggle to speak, or possibly to the presence of hemiplegia.

Lomas et al. (1989), in reporting on their development of the Communicative Effectiveness Index (CETI), which measures functional communication of the aphasic patient, also reviewed some of the literature on spousal attitudes toward the aphasic patient. Those authors noted some discrepancies in agreement about impairment between spouse (or significant other) and patient, and between speech–language pathologist and spouse.

Santo Pietro and Goldfarb (1995) reviewed an investigation done by Gordon-Adams (1985) on the self-reported behaviors and perceptions of wives of aphasic adults. The findings included the following:

1. resignation

2. avoidance of painful issues

3. resentment of new authority in the household and fear of new responsibility

4. enjoyment of new authority and reluctance to surrender it to a rehabilitated patient

5. focus on the patient's problems rather than on the caretaker's own problems or on solutions to the problems

6. infantilization of the patient

7. feelings of uniqueness and isolation

8. difficulty in discussing sexual problems

9. difficulties due to lack of understanding of aphasia, such as (a) perception that the patient is mentally incompetent or doesn't try hard enough, (b) idea that the patient's ability to use stereotypical responses is a good prognosis for language recovery, (c) intolerance and shock at the patient's use of profanity or of paraphasia, such as substitution of "mom" for "wife"

10. interpretation of intermittency of a patient's language competence as willfulness

Home Treatment by Caretakers

Home treatment by caretakers can be very effective if conducted under the proper conditions. Marshall et al. (1989) found that carefully monitored and trained (by speech–language pathologists) nonprofessionals can provide effective home treatment for the aphasic patient. To help put into effect what Marshall et al. found, Santo Pietro and Goldfarb (1995) suggested a number of "do's" and "don'ts" for caretakers of aphasic patients. These suggestions are meant to help overcome many of the problems mentioned above.

DOs for Caretakers:

we talk to infants / they even though do not understand

1. Do keep talking to the patient.

2. Do get the patient's attention before speaking.

3. Do talk slowly, to allow the patient time to process your message.

4. Do use short, one-idea, easy-to-process sentences.

5. Do establish the context of your message before you begin to expand on it (e.g., say, "Let's talk about tonight's supper" before starting a discussion of whether you should eat at home or go to a restaurant).

— this is patient specific and comes w/experience

6. Do give aphasic patients time to formulate what they want to say.

7. Do be an attentive listener and look for cues in the patient's tone of voice, facial expressions, and behavior to help you comprehend the message.

8. Do be empathetic and not sympathetic (e.g., say, "I am aware of how frustrated you must feel," not "Oh, you poor thing!").

9. Do adjust the communication schedule to the best time of day.

10. Do attend to any additional communication problems the patient may have along with the aphasia (e.g., hearing and visual difficulties, medication needs).

hearing aids dentures

11. Do allow the patient access to activity in the house and in the world.

12. Do allow the patient to continue any chores or responsibilities that remain manageable (e.g., gardening, caring for pets, cleaning).

13. Do foster success whenever possible. If the patient says or does something well (e.g., saying a name, dressing, answering the phone), be generous with your praise.

DON'Ts for Caretakers:

Can I give you the word?

1. Don't finish the patient's sentences unless the patient wants it.

2. Don't cut the patient off or interrupt when he or she is speaking. This may cause the aphasic patient to lose his or her train of thought.

3. Don't "fill in" the silence. The patient may need that time to process.

4. Don't turn your face away from the aphasic patient when you are speaking. The patient may need facial cues to help comprehend what you are saying.

Some thing will be easy for you and some things harder. Need to know what is what

Aphasia ❧ 95

5. Don't "talk down" to the aphasic patient. The patient will become highly sensitive to metalinguistic messages and will be insulted and "turned off" if you appear condescending.

6. Don't say things you do not want the aphasic patient to hear, assuming he or she will not understand. Quite often, he or she will.

7. Don't talk about the patient as if he or she were not here or were already dead (e.g., "He used to be a brilliant architect").

8. Don't talk only about activities of daily living.

9. Don't eliminate such activities as the theater, music, restaurants, and sporting events from the patient's daily lifestyle. All of us need stimulation, restoration for the soul, and fun in life to maximize and enhance communication.

10. Don't allow the aphasic patient to become isolated. Communication is a social undertaking.

Conversational Partners

In an approach called "conducting conversation," Boles (1998) reported on the success of including the spouse in aphasia treatment. When conversing with her husband (the aphasia patient), the spouse was instructed by a speech–language pathologist to reduce her speaking rate (fewer words per minute), reduce her percentage of talking turns, and to make fewer topic shifts. Discourse data taken after 2 weeks, 3 weeks, and 4 months showed that the patient had a successful increase in words per minute and talking turns, and fewer breakdowns in conversation.

Recently, Oelschlaeger (1999) reported on the participation of a conversation partner in the word searches of a person with aphasia. Thirty-eight videotaped conversational sequences from eight naturally occurring conversations of one couple were analyzed. Results showed that participation was determined by interactional techniques (e.g., direct or downward gaze) and interactional resources (e.g., information derived from the partners' shared life experience). The author provided examples of the successful use of interactional techniques and resources and their clinical implications.

A Final Note

Occasionally, a caretaker will tell the speech–language pathologist what sort of speech therapy the patient needs. The suggested therapy usually centers around the patient's oral expression. This happens when the clinician decides at the beginning of therapy, or after exhaustive amounts of therapy for oral expression deficit have not worked, to concentrate on the other modalities.

Speech–language pathologists should explain to the caretaker (and even doctors, nurses, etc., who think the same way) that working on the patient's oral expression would not be beneficial, whereas bolstering the other modalities would be more helpful. Apparently, to some caretakers and other health professionals, oral expression is the only way in which language is measured. When they hear the patient speak, it's like an instant assessment of normalcy. Clinicians know differently and must explain this to the caretaker and others.

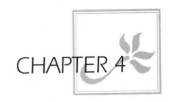

CHAPTER 4

Communication Disorders Associated with Right Hemisphere Damage

Definition

Right hemisphere damage (RHD) can cause problems in cognition, communication, or both. Problems in cognition would include the areas of attention, perception, orientation (time, place, and person), neglect, constructional impairment, anosognosia, prosopagnosia, and confabulation. Problems in communication would include the areas of language (particularly the semantic and pragmatic components) and speech (particularly the prosody component). Many times deficits in cognition can lead to deficits in language.

Symptoms

Cognition Deficits

(For a definition and discussion of the terms attention, perception, and orientation, see Chapters 1, 5, and 6).

Neglect
Neglect is defined as a failure to report, respond, or orient to novel or meaningful stimuli presented to the side opposite to a brain lesion, that

cannot be attributed to either an elemental sensory or motor defect (Filley & Kelly, 1990; Heilman, 1994). Severe neglect is more frequently associated with right than with left hemisphere lesions (Mesulam, 1990). Most patients with neglect have lesions of the parietal lobe, but neglect can also be associated with lesions of the frontal lobe, the cingulate gyrus (part of the limbic lobe or system), the temporal lobe, and the thalamus. The diseases that can cause neglect include stroke, tumors, trauma and degenerative disorders, or any condition that can damage the right hemisphere.

The neuropsychological mechanisms that have been assumed to account for neglect include disorders of attention (Hugdahl, Wester, & Asbjornsen, 1991; Robertson et al., 1994), motor intention-exploration (Heilman et al., 1985, as reported by Benson & Ardila, 1996), and spatial representations (perception) (Chieffi, Carlomagno, Silveri, & Gainotti, 1989; Gutbrod, Cohen, Maier, & Maier, 1987). Neglect can occur through the visual, auditory, tactile, or olfactory modality, singly or in combination, with the visual modality being the most frequently affected.

Myers (1994) has noted that left hemispatial neglect can cause visual, auditory, and communication problems. Visual problems are manifested when the patient, while viewing things on the left side, disrupts or omits the following: drawing, connecting dots, filling in states on a map, setting a clock, eating food from a tray, and attending to people in a room. Auditory problems on the patient's left side are shown by the patient's ignoring a ringing phone, people talking, or a bell or buzzer sounding. Communication problems are evident when the patient has left-sided problems in reading, and in spelling and punctuation when writing. For example, Stemmer, Giroux, & Joanette (1994) found that RHD subjects were deficient in the production and evaluation of requests when compared to control subjects. The authors postulated that attention and visuospatial abilities could cause the deficiencies. According to Benson and Ardila (1996), the reading problem can be called a neglect alexia or a spatial alexia, and the writing problem a spatial agraphia.

Constructional Impairment

Constructional impairment is quite common with both left hemisphere damaged (LHD) and right hemisphere damaged (RHD) patients. Due to problems in attention, perception, and neglect, the RHD patient will have difficulty in drawing or copying geometric designs (e.g., Benowitz, Moya, & Levine, 1990), reproducing stick figures, creating designs with colored blocks, or reproducing three-dimensional con-structions using wooden blocks. The RHD patient's reproductions will reflect a distorted and disorganized arrangement, whereas the LHD patient will show a primitive type of arrangement, but very much like the model. Swindell, Holland, Fromm, & Greenhouse (1988) found that when drawing a person, the LHD patients could make drawings that looked like a person and included appropriate facial characteristics, whereas the RHD patients made drawings that were disjointed and contained inappropriate characteristics.

Anosognosia and Prosopagnosia

Patients with right hemisphere damage can exhibit the cognitive defi-cits of anosognosia and prosopagnosia.

Anosognosia is an abnormal condition characterized by a real or feigned ability to perceive a defect, especially paralysis, on one side of the body, possibly attributable to a lesion in the right parietal lobe of the brain (Mosby Medical, Nursing, and Allied Health Dictionary, 1994). The individual may deny the existence of the affected part or may feel a depersonalization toward the affected part of the body. The condition may be associated with confabulation, inattention, or disturbed orien-tation of the body schema.

Prosopagnosia is an inability to recognize faces, even one's own face (Taber's Cyclopedic Medical Dictionary, 1997). The individual will rec-ognize persons they know by other features such as sound of voice, stride, body weight and size, or clothing. The condition is attributable to a lesion in the right temporal-occipital area of the brain.

Confabulation

The patient with right hemisphere damage typically will show few or no problems in auditory and reading comprehension, or in oral and written expression, as the adult aphasic patient would (e.g., Cappa, Papagno, & Vallar, 1990). The RHD patient might show irrelevant lan-guage where the response does not relate to the stimulus or contains confabulations (the fabrication of experiences or situations, often recounted in a detailed and plausible way, to fill in and cover up gaps in the memory, apparently without any intent to deceive), and/or prop-agation (an increased amount of irrelevant language that many times connects or includes mention of the patient's illness and its relation to the environment, in an erroneous manner).

Hough (1990) found that RHD patients confabulated more and strayed more from a central theme than did LHD patients and persons without brain damage. Sohlberg and Ehlhardt (1998) have noted that, based on observations of behavior, confabulation can be classified as spontaneous or provoked. Spontaneous confabulations are uttered without apparent incitement and are often fantastic or implausible. Provoked confabulations tend to happen as a reaction to questioning and often are tied to some real event. Additional information on confabulation and propagation can be found in Chapter 6.

As an example of confabulation, one RHD patient responded to this author's inquiry as to whether he did his assignment in the following manner: The patient explained that he was unable to do the assignment because he was ill with a toothache all weekend and had to see a dentist, whom he identified as this author. He further indicated that his sole complaint and the reason he continued to see this author were problems with his teeth. A conversation with family members revealed that his teeth were in fact in very good shape and that he had neither required a dentist nor complained of a toothache for quite some time.

Communication Deficits

Language Abilities

A sampling of studies reveals that the RHD patient can have difficulty with drawing inferences (implied information), abstract words, story arrangement, comprehension of spoken narrative discourse, and pragmatic abilities.

Inferences. Brownell, Potter, Bihrle, & Gardner (1986) found that RHD patients were deficient in inferential reasoning, and Brownell, Simpson, Bihrle, Potter, & Gardner (1990) observed that the appreciation of metaphoric and nonmetaphoric alternative meanings of single words was impaired in RHD subjects. McDonald and Wales (1986) found that RHD patients did more poorly than the control group in processing inferences.

Myers and Brookshire (1996) found that 24 RHD subjects, particularly those with high levels of neglect, were significantly impaired relative to the 30 non–brain-damaged (NBD) subjects in generating accurate inferences from pictures, but not in their ability to recognize and identify pictured elements.

Tompkins, Bloise, Timko, & Baumgartner (1994) observed that 25 RHD and 25 LHD subjects showed deficiencies in working memory and tasks requiring inference revision; the RHD group especially with the task that involved the most demanding comprehension processes. No meaningful association within the above conditions was observed for normally aging subjects.

Winner, Brownell, Happe, Blum, & Pincus (1998) found that 13 RHD patients performed worse than 20 normal control subjects when asked to distinguish lies from jokes, confirming their known difficulty with discourse interpretation.

On the other hand, a few other studies indicated different results. Tompkins (1990) found that RHD subjects performed similarly to LHD and normal control subjects in the automatic condition (discouraging the use of any associative strategies) and when provided with specific processing strategies, indicating that they retained some knowledge of metaphoric word meanings. When left to glean strategies for themselves, both brain-damaged groups had difficulty. In another study, Tompkins, Boada, & McGarry (1992) observed that no significant differences existed in the processing of familiar idioms between normally aging, RHD, and LHD groups.

Abstract and concrete words. Goulet and Joanette (1994) found that in a sentence completion task requiring abstract or concrete words, the use of both kinds of words was more impaired in RHD than in normal subjects.

Story arrangement. Schneiderman, Murasugi, and Saddy (1992) observed that RHD subjects had more difficulty with story arrangement than did LHD and NBD subjects.

Comprehension of spoken narrative discourse. Using an earlier version of their *Discourse Comprehension Test* (see Chapter 3), Nicholas and Brookshire (1995a) found that in the comprehension of spoken narrative discourse, 20 RHD subjects had more correct responses when questions assessed main ideas than when they assessed details, and more correct responses when questions assessed stated information than when they assessed implied information. In addition, stated information had stronger effects on their comprehension of details than on their comprehension of main ideas.

Pragmatic abilities. Several studies have shown that RHD subjects are deficient in their pragmatic abilities (Bloom, Borod, Obler, & Gerstman, 1993; Foldi, 1987; Kaplan, Brownell, Jacobs, & Gardner,

1990). As an example of a breakdown in pragmatic behavior (not maintaining proper decorum in a communicative setting), one RHD patient responded to the direction, "Tell me three things every good citizen should do" in the following manner: "Go to sleep, get up, and take a good ____" (the third item can best be described as a bodily function performed in the bathroom). The patient was so pleased with himself for giving that answer that he proceeded to laugh and act jolly for the next few minutes of the session.

Speech Abilities

Prosody. Prosody is a component of speech production that includes such features as intonation, stress, rate, rhythm, melody, pitch, volume, spacing between words, and intervals and pauses in conversation, all of which can convey linguistic and emotional (or affective) (e.g., happy, sad, angry, shocked, gloating, neutral) information. The effects of prosody also involve the listener's comprehension of the linguistic and emotional information provided by the speaker.

Comprehension and expression of emotional speech. In her review, Myers (1994) noted that RHD patients may have difficulty in comprehending and expressing emotional speech. Studies have not made it clear whether this emotional inappropriateness is a result of an emotional (or affective) disorder, or of a more general attention deficit that reduces responsiveness to the external environment.

Reduced responsiveness may impede the understanding of extralinguistic cues (facial expression, body language, gestures, and prosody) from which one can infer the emotional atmosphere of situations and narratives. Borod et al. (1989) found that the "flat affect" of schizophrenics most resembled that of RHD subjects (choices included Parkinson's subjects [hypokinetic dysarthria] and normal subjects). Perceptual problems in spatial judgment and feature integration may also contribute to a reduction in the ability to recognize emotional facial expression.

Comprehension of emotional (or affective) prosody is tested by having the subject listen to neutral sentences expressed with an emotional overlay, and then identify the mood of the speaker.

Comprehension and expression of linguistic information. RHD can also produce deficits in prosodic *comprehension* and *expression* of linguistic information. Comprehension of linguistic prosody is tested by having the subject listen to prosodic features used to convey (a) different types of sentences (e.g., declarative, interrogative, or exclamatory), (b) different word meanings through use of emphatic stress (e.g., distinguishing "greenhouse" from "green house," and (c) linguistic stress markers that can alter sentence meanings (e.g., "John wants the **red** bike" versus "**John** wants the red bike").

Then again, comprehension difficulties in prosody may be tied to impaired tonal perception and to impaired attention. All in all, studies in RHD prosodic comprehension are not clear on whether the problem is caused by a linguistic, emotional, or cognitive (perception, attention) disturbance.

In his review, Duffy (1995) noted that aprosodia are prosodic impairments in the *interpretation* or *production* of speech that may be uniquely associated with right hemisphere damage. In the production of speech, prosody disturbances may be associated with various lesion sites (e.g., frontal lobe, frontoparietal lobes, and subcortical areas), motor speech disorders (e.g., dysarthria, apraxia of speech), and cognitive and affective deficits (e.g., depression).

The aprosodic speech pattern is often described as flat, indifferent, devoid of expression and emotion, having little spontaneous prosody, computer-like or robotic, monotonous, and lacking the ability to modulate the voice to convey the subtleties of language (e.g., irony, sarcasm). Duffy (1995) also noted that studies of aprosodia have yielded mixed results, and the defining characteristics and nature of the problem underlying aprosodia are still not well understood.

Communication abilities and inference impairment. Myers (1994) has postulated that most of the language problems of the RHD patient are due to an inference impairment. She defined an inference as a hypothesis about sensory data where that input is not only sensed but also interpreted. Inferences depend on the following processes: (a) attention to individual cues, (b) selection of relevant cues, (c) integration of relevant cues with one another, and (d) association of cues with prior experience.

Myers (1994) further noted that this underlying inference impairment leads to disturbances in the following areas: (a) producing informative content (e.g., RHD patients may produce a lot of words, but much of it is empty speech), (b) integrating narrative information (e.g., RHD patients may lose the gist of what they hear and subsequently what they say), (c) generating alternative meanings (e.g., RHD patients will have problems with understanding figurative language such as metaphors, idioms, and proverbs; irony; sarcasm; humor; a person's motives), (d) comprehending and expressing emotion, and (e) comprehending and producing prosody.

Etiology

The types of focal brain lesions that cause adult aphasia are the same ones that can cause right hemisphere damage. These include cerebrovascular accidents, trauma to the brain, and brain tumors as the major causes. The lesser causes include abscesses, infectious diseases, and degenerative diseases of the brain.

Diagnosis

Diagnostic procedures for determining the communication disorders associated with right hemisphere damage can involve (a) establishing background information, (b) giving a neurologic evaluation, (c) employing informal tests, and (d) employing formal tests.

Establishing Background Information and the Neurologic Evaluation

These procedures can be found at the beginning of the "Diagnosis" section of Chapter 3.

Informal Tests

Cognition Deficits

The participants involved in the diagnosis of *neglect* can include the neurologist, the neuropsychologist, the occupational therapist, and the speech–language pathologist. The speech–language pathologist can get a good idea as to whether neglect is present by doing the following: (a) for visual neglect, asking the patient to draw symmetrical items (clock, figure and face of a human, baseball diamond, football field, connecting dots, filling in a map), and perform reading and writing tasks; (b) for auditory neglect, standing behind the patient and presenting auditory commands (e.g., "Pick up the pencil," "Look at the window," "Snap your fingers," "Tap the table") of equal intensity to each ear.

General observation of the patient's reaching for items, pointing to things, applying lipstick, results of shaving, and wearing of eyeglasses can also be used for determining neglect. The informal diagnosis of neglect is warranted if the patient misses or distorts any or all of the items presented to the left side.

Facial affect can be assessed by having the patient produce a variety of facial expressions on command (e.g., happy, sad, angry, shocked, afraid, neutral). The clinician can produce a variety of facial expressions and then have the patient tell what they represent.

Communication Deficits

Prosody can be tested by having the patient say or listen to inherently neutral sentences (e.g., saying, "Today is Wednesday," or listening to that sentence and producing or recognizing a happy, sad, angry, shocked, neutral, etc. quality). Bloom, Borod, Obler, & Gerstman (1992) observed that RHD subjects had a selective impairment in producing emotional contents. Tompkins (1991a) found that in automatic and effortful processing of emotional intonation, the RHD subjects were slower than LHD subjects.

Pragmatic abilities can be checked by noting the patient's eye contact, topic maintenance, turn-taking, loudness level, awareness of errors, attention, etc. Bloom et al. (1993) found that emotional content suppressed pragmatic performance among RHD subjects. Kaplan et al. (1990) observed that RHD individuals were more deficient in picking up pragmatic cues than were matched control subjects.

Language deficits can be evaluated by using any of the tests noted later in this chapter, or by using selected portions of the aphasia batteries mentioned in the "Diagnosis" section of Chapter 3. Questions probing orientation to time, place, and person, and general information can be added (see the "Diagnosis" section of Chapter 5).

One RHD patient, a lawyer and former foreign diplomat attached to his country's mission at the United Nations, had an excellent vocabulary in English. He could give fine definitions of single words and talk about some of his experiences at the UN (this author is not sure if they were true or not). His problems became apparent when he was asked to respond to time, place, and person orientation stimuli (e.g., "What year (season, month, day of the week) is it?" "What is today's date?" "Where do you live?" "Who do you live with?" "Where are you right now?" The patient's responses were off not by 1 year, 1 month, or 1 day, but by as much as 10 years, 6 months, or 3 days. He had no concept of where he lived or how long he had lived there, nor could he identify family members. He also exhibited neglect, flat affect, and pragmatic problems in eye contact, turn-taking, and topic maintenance.

To ascertain if the patient digresses (e.g., confabulations) or can integrate ideas, the clinician can ask open-ended questions such as defining proverbs, telling three things that every good citizen should do, defining words, responding to items requiring a sequence of events (e.g., "What would you do if you saw smoke?" "How would you fry an egg?" "How did you get to work?" "What did your workday consist of?" "How do you wash your hair?").

Picture descriptions can be used for evaluating the patient's narrative verbal output. Myers (1994) describes a procedure whereby narrative verbal output is broken down into interpretive and literal concepts. An interpretive score is arrived at by dividing the total number of concepts by the number of interpretive concepts. Examples are given of interpretive and literal concepts, and data are cited on how non–brain-damaged and RHD patients performed using this analysis. The non–brain-damaged subjects produced almost twice as many interpretive responses as the RHD subjects.

Formal Tests

Cognitive and language abilities can be tested with some of the batteries available for testing the RHD patient. Adamovich and Brooks (1981) described a procedure for testing the communicative abilities of RHD patients. They borrowed portions of tests used in aphasia, visual organization, and learning aptitude.

The Discourse Comprehension Test (Brookshire & Nicholas, 1997) assesses both listening and reading comprehension (see Chapter 3, "Diagnosis").

The Evaluation of Communication Problems in Right Hemisphere Dysfunction (Burns, Halper, & Mogil, 1985) and the *RIC Evaluation of Communication Problems in Right Hemisphere Dysfunction* (RICE–R) (Halper,

Cherney, Burns, & Mogil, 1996, cited in Golper & Cherney, 1999) offer protocols for evaluating the RHD patient by (a) interviewing the patient; (b) observing the patient in contact with hospital staff and family members; (c) evaluating attention, eye contact, awareness of illness, orientation to time, place, and person, facial expression, intonation, and topic maintenance; (d) tests of visual scanning and tracking; (e) evaluating written expression; (f) rating pragmatic skills; and (g) a language test using metaphors.

The Mini Inventory of Right Brain Injury (MIRBI) (Pimental & Kingsbury, 1989) assesses (a) visual scanning; (b) integrity of gnosis (e.g., object identification); (c) integrity of body image; (d) reading and writing; (e) serial sevens (e.g., subtracting 7 from 100, subtracting 7 from the remainder, and so on); (f) integrity of praxis (e.g., drawing a clock); (g) speech intonation; (h) humor, incongruities, absurdities, figurative language, and similarities; (i) affect; and (j) general behavior.

The Right Hemisphere Language Battery (RHLB) (Bryan, 1989) evaluates (a) comprehension of spoken metaphors, (b) comprehension of printed metaphors, (c) comprehension of inferred meaning (reading), (d) appreciation of humor (reading), (e) pointing to picture by name, (f) production of emphatic stress in spoken sentences, and (g) discourse analysis of spontaneous conversation.

The Ross Information Processing Assessment (RIPA–2) (Ross-Swain, 1996) assesses the following 10 areas of communicative and cognitive functioning: (a) immediate memory, (b) recent memory, (c) temporal orientation (recent memory), (d) temporal orientation (remote memory), (e) spatial orientation, (f) orientation to environment, (g) recall of general information, (h) problem solving and abstract reasoning, (i) organization, and (j) auditory processing and retention.

Therapy

The first goal of therapy is to inform the patient and the caretaker(s) about the nature and the consequences of the disorder.

The RHD patient can have problems in the processes of attention, perception, neglect, constructional abilities, emotions, inference abilities, prosody, and pragmatic functioning. Cognitive impairment could lead to overall mild language problems and to the specific irrelevant language errors (confabulations and propagations) displayed by the patient.

Although not as clearly delineated as with the aphasia patient, spontaneous recovery (and prognosis) in the RHD patient can show many of the same patterns. In spontaneous recovery for the RHD patient, the major emphasis would be on the retrieval of the nonlanguage functions described in the previous paragraph, and the minor emphasis would be on the overall mild language problems (see the "Spontaneous Recovery" section in Chapter 3).

With prognosis (see the "Prognosis" section in Chapter 3), the indicators most applicable to the RHD patient would be age, time of entering therapy, neurologic damage, will to improve and acceptance of limitations, family attitude and encouragement, initial evaluation, length and intensity of therapy, and physical condition.

In reaction to their illness, RHD patients can often show anosognosia, which is defined as a lack of awareness, denial, or a tendency to minimize the condition. They can often be overly optimistic and jocular, and at the same time exhibit a lack of motivation. They may also have unrealistic goals (e.g., going back to work); have time, place, and person disorientation; fail to recognize familiar faces; and have grooming deficits. They can be impulsive and have difficulty in getting to or understanding the main point in conversation.

Due to many of the reactions listed above (e.g., overly optimistic, unrealistic goals, jocularity, minimizing the illness) and the mild language problem that can occur, families tend to believe the patient. This belief in a false, rosy picture, coupled with their own hopes for a return to normalcy, can lead to a very unrealistic perception of the patient's true capabilities.

The second goal of therapy is to provide the appropriate treatment approaches and techniques.

Efficacy of Therapy for the Communication Disorders Associated with Right Hemisphere Damage

Efficacy of treatment studies for communication disorders associated with right hemisphere damage are difficult to find in the literature. One possible reason is that the symptoms of RHD are not, relatively speaking, as clear-cut as the symptoms of adult aphasia. In aphasia, the symptoms involve a language breakdown, and all efforts in diagnosis and treatment are concentrated in that one area.

The symptoms in RHD can involve problems in attention, perception, neglect, constructional abilities, emotion, inference ability, prosody, language, and in particular the pragmatic aspects of language. Because of the variety of symptoms, diagnosis and treatment are geared not only toward language but to cognitive and behavioral problems as well.

There is now some question whether RHD patients are best treated by the relatively long-time use of the treatment of symptoms approach, or by a relatively new, alternative, treatment of cause approach (to help the symptoms). For example, emotion can be treated with techniques that directly correct the patient's recognition and production of flat affect (emotion).

As an alternative approach to correcting the symptoms of emotion, Myers (1994) proposed using items designed to increase patient abilities to generate alternative meanings and integrate information. In her opinion, emotional deficits arise from the same source as narrative-level deficits, namely, an underlying inference impairment.

The two types of research design that are used to determine the efficacy of treatment in aphasia can be used with the RHD population (see the "Efficacy of Aphasia Therapy" section in Chapter 3).

Several programs of treatment (described later in this chapter) have been identified as being useful by Anderson and Miller (1986), Brookshire (1997), Burns et al. (1985), Myers (1994), Santo Pietro and Goldfarb (1995), and Tompkins (1995). They include treatment for the following: attention, perception, and neglect problems; constructional impairment; emotional and prosody impairment; pragmatic impairment, integrating information (inference); time, place, and person orientation; anosognosia; prosopagnosia; and general memory deficits.

Therapy for Attention, Perception, and Neglect Problems

Anderson and Miller (1986), Brookshire (1997), Burns et al. (1985), and Tompkins (1995) have suggested many of the following tasks:

1. Clinician should sit on patient's right, move gradually to his or her left, and say to patient, "Look at me."

2. As a self-cueing strategy, patient is taught to say, "Look to the left."

In items 3 through 24, the clinician asks the patient to perform the listed task.

3. Look to the right, left, right visual field.

4. Point to objects in the room in his or her right and then left visual field.

5. Name pictures of people, objects, and food moving from his or her right to left; starting with large items and moving to smaller items.

6. Name body parts in the right and then the left visual field.

7. Touch objects in the left visual field and then name them.

8. Listen to bell (behind patient, first on right and then on left side) and then reach for it.

9. Listen to clinician's voice (behind patient, first on right and then on left side) and then point to source.

10. Listen for a specific word within a group of words (spoken in front of and then behind patient, first on right and then on left side).

11. Identify voice and color of clothing of person in left visual field.

12. Look at door on his or her left and count the number of people coming in.

13. Watch TV placed to his or her left.

14. Label body parts in pictures (e.g., left leg, right hand).

15. Answer questions about a calendar, especially its left side.

16. Find locations on left, using a map or busy picture.

17. Read single words, phrases, sentences, and paragraphs on left; this task moves from large to small print, and from concrete to abstract material. Chieffi et al. (1989) found that in lexical comprehension, aphasic subjects failed because of semantic discrimination, whereas the RHD subjects failed because of perceptual discrimination.

18. Scan or sort objects, pictures, or words according to shape, meaning, color, category, and function.

19. Scan or sort alphabet or number tiles, cubes, pictures.

20. Set a clock with movable hands to different times.

21. Do arithmetic that requires columns.

22. Work simple to complex puzzles (e.g., jigsaw, crossword).

23. Follow up and down columns in newspapers.

24. Play easy card games, tic-tac-toe, checkers.

25. Clinician arranges numbers, letters, pictures, and objects in a certain way and then removes them. Patient has to duplicate arrangement.

26. Patient is asked to remember letters, numbers, forms, and words and to write them.

27. Clinician discusses with patient the visual items that need remembering (e.g., writing down times for breakfast, lunch, dinner, therapy, other appointments).

28. Patient is asked to describe from memory what has just been seen in a picture.

Therapy for Constructional Impairment

Tasks designed to help the patient overcome his or her constructional impairment are as follows:

1. Patient is asked to draw lines from A to B to C, etc. on a paper or a blackboard.

2. Patient is asked to bisect lines that are placed at different angles randomly on a page.

3. Patient is asked to connect the dots to form letters, words, or shapes (see Santo Pietro and Goldfarb, 1995, for examples).

4. Patient is asked to trace a line straight across a page. Then he or she practices writing words and then sentences, keeping

them on the line. Patient also uses graph paper for writing words and sentences.

5. Patient is asked to copy simple drawings (e.g., stick figures, geometric forms). It is useful to have the original drawing on lined or graph paper and to ask the patient to copy on the same kind of paper. This will help the patient check for the correct spatial orientation.

6. Patient is asked to draw a daisy, clock, person, etc., including the left half.

7. Patient is shown simple drawings of people, objects, shapes, etc., and asked to draw them after they have been removed.

Therapy for Time, Place, and Person Orientation

Burns et al. (1985) proposed instructing the patient in most of the following areas for biographical and environmental information, and for estimating time intervals:

1. patient's name

2. year, month, day, date, time of day

3. present location

4. home address (number, street, section, borough, town, city, state, county)

5. home phone number

6. significant family members' names and pertinent data (e.g., married or single, number of children, number of grand-children)

7. reason for hospitalization

8. names of the president and vice-president of the U.S., governor of state, mayor of city or town, two U.S. senators from home state

9. estimated time intervals for getting out of bed and turning off alarm, brushing teeth, showering, putting on makeup or shaving, getting dressed, eating breakfast

Therapy for Anosognosia (Lack of Awareness of Illness and Deficits)

Procedures designed to help the patient overcome his or her lack of awareness of the illness and deficits are as follows:

1. Clinician informs patient as to what they're working on and why (e.g., "You're not paying attention to anyone who is on your left side.").

2. Clinician informs patient in a gentle manner when he or she denies the impairments.

3. Clinician provides a lot of enthusiastic, positive feedback to patient because awareness information and training might be perceived as negative.

4. Clinician counsels patient's family about anosognosia (e.g., patient might convince family that nothing is wrong).

Therapy for Prosopagnosia (Facial Recognition Impairment)

Burns et al. (1985) suggested the following procedures for helping the patient to recognize individuals. The clinician simultaneously presents photographs and brief audio recordings (if possible). The patient has to name the person, and the following cues can be used:

1. male or female?

2. adult or child?

3. hair color?

4. body size?

5. Distinguishing facial features (e.g., scar, size or shape of nose, beard, eye color, voice characteristics, including accent, dialect, habitual use of word or phrase)?

Therapy for General Memory Deficits

If needed, see suggestions for memory deficits noted in Chapters 5 and 6.

Therapy for Integrating Information

Anderson and Miller (1986), Burns et al. (1985), and Tompkins (1995) have proposed many of the following tasks:

1. Clinician helps patient to understand the daily routine involving medication times and their importance, food selections, etc.

2. Clinician helps patient to understand conversations with other professionals (doctors, nurses, etc.).

    In items 3 through 11, the clinician asks the patient to perform the listed task.

3. Tell a story that has sequential events (e.g., making scrambled eggs). Roman, Brownell, Potter, Seibold, & Gardner (1987) found that RHD patients have a relatively well-preserved ("script") knowledge. Scripts represent knowledge of the sequence of events in familiar situations (e.g., washing one's hair would involve the following: turning on the water, wetting the hair, applying the shampoo, rinsing, drying, etc.). The familiarity of the sequence of events in frequently occurring situations allows one to make inferences about information that is not directly stated in discourse.

4. Read or listen to a story and then summarize it or answer questions about it (e.g., important newspaper and magazine articles, TV stories). Nicholas and Brookshire (1995a) suggested the use of scripts, and main idea and stated information strength as a means of enhancing discourse comprehension.

5. Relate or write a description of a picture, including any emotions portrayed by the picture.

6. Put words into groupings (e.g., five fruits, five cities).

7. Relate what proverbs or analogies mean (e.g., *once in a blue moon; Don't cry over spilled milk*).

8. Relate how one would get to particular locations (e.g., in current facility, former workplace, well-known landmarks).

9. Figure out, itemize, and arrange charts, graphs, checkbooks, calendars.

10. Figure out arithmetic problems that are given in story form.

11. Read or listen to a controversial story and take a stand on it (e.g., capital punishment, abortion rights, dropping of atom bomb). Rehak et al. (1992) found that RHD patients were strongly influenced by interest level in their ability to process a story.

Santo Pietro and Goldfarb (1995) offer additional items for integrating information. For these items, the clinician asks the patient to do the following:

1. respond to specified and implied information (e.g., *The boss fired the man for being late. Why did the boss fire the man? Why was the man late?*)

2. explain metaphors (e.g., *She's the toast of the town.*)

3. explain similes (e.g., *She's as American as apple pie.*)

4. rephrase figurative language (e.g., *He saw red.*)

The following four examples of understanding inferences were developed by Fuchs (1981) and elaborated on by Santo Pietro and Goldfarb (1995):

1. Laura had a stomach virus. She ate nothing for 3 days.

   A. Did Laura have a stomach virus? Did Laura have a sore throat?

   B. Did Laura lose weight? Did Laura gain weight?

2. The teacher bit into the juicy apple. She enjoyed her afternoon snack.

   A. Did the teacher bite into a fruit? Did the teacher bite into a vegetable?

   B. Did the teacher bite into a juicy apple? Did the teacher bite into a dry apple?

3. Barbara swept the kitchen floor. Now it was nice and clean.

   A. Did Barbara use a broom? Did Barbara use a sponge?

   B. Was the kitchen floor swept? Was the bedroom floor swept?

4. The student studied hard for the test. She slept poorly the night before.

   A. Did the student sleep poorly? Did the student sleep soundly?

   B. Did the student feel anxious about the test? Did the student feel confident about the test?

Example one is an inference made through *consequence,* whereby subsequent actions or states of being are suggested by an event or series of events. One can infer that Laura lost weight due to the stomach virus and consequent failure to eat for 3 days.

Example two is an inference made through *semantic entailment,* whereby the listener knows that statements valid for the member element may also be valid for the class in general. One can infer that the teacher bit into a fruit because an apple is a member of the general category called fruits.

Example three is an inference made through *implied instrument,* whereby tools, containers, vehicles, or other objects are conceptually necessitated by the function or operation of certain verbs. One can infer that Barbara used a broom from the use of the verb *swept.*

Example four is an inference made through *presupposition,* whereby prior actions or states of being are suggested by an event or series of events. One can infer that the student felt anxious about the test because sleeping poorly the night before the exam can be a symptom of anxiety.

Therapy for Pragmatic Impairment

Brookshire (1997) has noted that eye contact, turn-taking, and topic maintenance are often treated because they are relatively manageable, and their improvement can have quite an effect on the patient's appropriate use of language. Eye contact is practiced by the clinician's saying to the patient, "Look at me" during conversations. This activity is then followed by an analysis of why it is important to maintain eye contact during conversation (e.g., shows interest, alertness, concentration, politeness, comprehension). Another procedure is to instruct the patient to make eye contact at the beginning and end of his or her own utterances and then to do the same with the utterances of his or her conversational partner. The beginning and end of utterances is a self-cueing device.

Turn-taking is treated by first discussing with the patient why turn-taking is important during conversation with others (e.g., hearing the full message, getting the meaning of the message, what interruptions do). The clinician then instructs the patient to watch videotapes of conversation between two or more persons (e.g., television, movies) and then analyze the turn-taking of the participants. Other techniques include having the patient write a simple script or engage in free conversation with the clinician and analyze the appropriate spots for turn-taking.

Topic maintenance is taught by reading stories in newspapers and magazines, watching videotapes of conversations involving two or more participants, and engaging in structured conversations. The above activities are performed together by the clinician and patient, with an analysis of when the topic is maintained and when it changes or stops.

Myers (1994) has stated that most of the language problems of the RHD patient are due to an inference impairment. She advocates treating the inference problem as a means of ameliorating the pragmatic impairment of the patient.

Therapy for Emotional and Prosody Impairment

There are no set guidelines in the literature for treating emotional and prosodic impairment. However, if a treatment by symptom approach is desired, portions of diagnostic material can be used as possible therapy techniques. For example, facial affect can be worked on by instructing the patient to produce a variety of facial expressions (e.g., happy, sad, angry, shocked, gloating, neutral). Prosody can be worked on by having the patient say or listen to inherently neutral sentences (e.g., saying or listening to "Today is Wednesday" and producing or recognizing a happy, sad, angry, shocked, neutral, etc. quality).

Before undertaking these therapy procedures, the clinician should make sure that the patient does not have a true emotional disorder. The clinician can recommend a psychiatrist or psychologist for help in this matter. Borod et al. (1989) found that the flat affect of schizophrenics resembled that of the RHD patient. Myers (1994) has advocated that training in the comprehension of other contextual cues is likely to be a more effective way of treating emotional and prosodic impairment. Tompkins (1991b) found that the redundancy of stimuli enhanced the emotional inferencing abilities of RHD and LHD adults.

The third goal of therapy is to encourage the patient and the caretaker(s) to continue the rehabilitative process outside of the clinical setting.

Although not as clearly delineated, home treatment by caretakers of RHD patients can benefit from many of the suggestions mentioned for the aphasia patient (see the "Home Treatment by Caretakers" section in Chapter 3). The most applicable suggestions for the RHD patient follow (numbering follows Chapter 3).

DOs for Caretakers:

1. Do keep talking to the patient.

2. Do get the patient's attention before speaking.

3. Do talk slowly, to allow the patient time to process your message.

4. Do use short, one-idea, easy-to-process sentences.

5. Do establish the context of your message before you begin to expand on it.

6. Do give the patient time to formulate what he or she wants to say.

7. Do be an attentive listener and look for cues in the patient's tone of voice, facial expressions, and behavior to help you comprehend the message.

8. Do be empathetic and not sympathetic.

9. Do adjust the communication schedule to the best time of day.

10. Do attend to any additional communication problems the patient may have.

11. Do allow the patient access to activity in the house and in the world.

12. Do allow the patient to continue any chores or responsibilities that remain manageable.

13. Do foster success whenever possible. If the patient says or does something well, be generous with your praise.

DON'Ts for Caretakers:

1. Don't finish the patient's sentences unless the patient wants it.

2. Don't cut the patient off or interrupt when he or she is speaking.

3. Don't "fill in" the silence. The patient may need that time to process.

4. Don't turn your face away from the patient. The patient may need facial cues to help him or her comprehend what you are saying.

5. Don't "talk down" to the patient.

6. Don't talk only about activities of daily living.

7. Don't eliminate such activities as the theater, music, restaurants, and sporting events from the patient's daily lifestyle.

8. Don't allow the patient to become isolated. Communication is a social undertaking.

Nicholas and Brookshire (1995a) recommended that the patient's communication partners be trained by the clinician to use a strategic approach to communication discourse. With the knowledge that RHD patients have strengths in scripts and main idea and stated information, the communication partner might be encouraged to clearly state the topic or theme early in the discourse. The communication partner can increase the main idea information by presenting it redundantly and connecting it to the theme or central points of the message. The central points of the message could be paraphrased and elaborated on, and then explained as to how they relate to the more peripheral details. Communication partners might be advised to provide important information in a stated (direct) manner, rather than requiring the patient to make inferences through implication. These strategies may be particularly worthwhile when the information to be understood is less familiar to the patient.

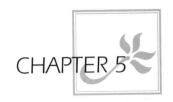

CHAPTER 5

Communication Disorders Associated with Dementia

Definition

In its definition, the *Diagnostic and Statistical Manual of Mental Disorders* (DSM–IV) (American Psychiatric Association, 1994) states that the essential feature of a dementia is the development of multiple cognitive deficits that include memory impairment and at least one of the following: aphasia, apraxia, agnosia, or a disturbance in executive functioning. The cognitive deficits must be sufficiently severe to cause impairment in occupational or social functioning (e.g., going to school, working, shopping, dressing, bathing, handling finances, and other activities of daily living) and must represent a decline from a previously higher level of functioning.

Symptoms and Etiology

The American Psychiatric Association (1994) describes the multiple cognitive deficits that can exist in dementia. They are presented below with some modifications.

Memory impairment is needed to make the diagnosis of a dementia and is a prominent early symptom (Cummings & Benson, 1992; note that in Pick's disease memory is preserved in the early and middle stages of the condition). Persons with dementia become impaired in their ability to learn new information, and/or they forget previously learned information. They may lose items like wallets and keys, forget food cooking on the stove, and become lost in unfamiliar neighborhoods. In the advanced stages, these individuals can forget their occupation, schooling, birthday, family members, and their own names. (See other parts of this chapter and Chapter 6 for additional comments on memory.)

Aphasia is a language disturbance that affects auditory and reading comprehension and oral and written expression, and can appear in persons with dementia. In the advanced stages of dementia, individuals may be mute or have a deteriorated speech pattern characterized by echolalia (echoing what is heard) or palilalia (repeating sounds or words over and over). (See Chapter 3 and other parts of this chapter for additional comments on aphasia.)

Apraxia is an impairment in the ability to execute motor activities despite intact motor abilities, sensory function, and understanding of the required task, and may appear in individuals with dementia. These persons will be impaired in their ability to pantomime the use of objects (e.g., brushing teeth) or to execute familiar motor acts (e.g., waving goodbye). Problems in cooking, dressing, and drawing may be attributed to apraxia.

Agnosia is a failure to recognize or identify objects despite intact sensory function, and can appear in persons with dementia. Individuals may have normal visual acuity but lose the ability to recognize objects such as pencils or chairs. In the latter stages, they may be unable to recognize family members or even themselves in the mirror. They may have normal tactile sensation but be unable to identify through touch, objects placed in their hands (e.g., pencil, coin, key).

Executive dysfunction is an impairment in the ability to think abstractly and to plan, initiate, sequence, monitor, and stop complex activities, and may appear in persons with dementia. Impairment in abstract thinking may be shown by difficulty coping with new or novel tasks or the avoidance of situations that require the processing of new and complex information.

Executive dysfunction is also apparent in the reduced ability to shift mental sets (e.g., moving from counting to saying the alphabet, then days of the week, then months of the year), to generate new or novel information (e.g., noting similarities and differences between a doctor and lawyer or a farmer and gardener, or naming as many animals as possible in one minute), or to execute serial motor activities (e.g., imitating simple tapping rhythms with the hand or using the telephone). Executive dysfunction can interfere with the activities of daily life (e.g., ability to work, plan activities, or budget finances). (See Chapters 1 and 6 for additional comments on executive dysfunction.)

Associated Features and Disorders

Associated features and disorders of dementia can include difficulty with spatial tasks (copying drawings); poor judgment and insight; little or no awareness of memory loss or other cognitive abnormalities; an unrealistic assessment of their own abilities and prognosis (e.g., planning to start a new business); an underestimation of risks involved in certain activities (e.g., driving); violence; suicidal tendencies; motor disturbances of gait; disinhibited behavior; neglecting personal hygiene; showing undue familiarity with strangers; disregarding conventional rules of social conduct; dysarthria; anxiety, mood, and sleep disturbances; delusions; hallucinations (mostly visual); delirium (acute confusional state); and a vulnerability to physical stressors (e.g., illness or minor surgery) and psychosocial stressors (e.g., going to hospital, bereavement) (American Psychiatric Association, 1994).

Age and Course

Depending on the etiology, dementia usually occurs late in life, with the greatest number of cases appearing in those above 85 years of age. Dementia may be progressive, static, or remitting. Historically, it implied a progressive or irreversible course, and this chapter will deal with patients who present that picture.

Types

Dementia is classified as cortical, subcortical, or mixed cortical-subcortical (Cummings & Benson, 1992). Cortical dementia has its major neuropathology in the cerebral cortex. Subcortical dementia has its major neuropathology in the basal ganglia, thalamus, and the brain stem. A mixed dementia has its major neuropathology in both cortical and subcortical structures.

Speech and language problems will vary typically according to the type of dementia. Cortical dementia is characterized by language disorders. Subcortical dementia features speech disorders. Mixed cortical-subcortical dementia presents both language and speech disorders (Benson & Ardila, 1996; Cummings & Benson, 1992).

Cortical Dementia

Alzheimer's Disease

The condition that typically produces a cortical dementia is Alzheimer's disease (AD), which comprises about 50% of all cases of dementia. The neuropathology in the brains of these patients includes *neuritic plaques, neurofibrillary tangles,* and *granulovacuolar degeneration* (Bayles, 1994; Cummings & Benson, 1992). Neuritic plaques are minute areas of tissue degeneration consisting of granular deposits and remnants of neuronal processes. Neurofibrillary tangles are filamentous structures in the nerve cell body, dendrites, axon, and synaptic endings, which become twisted or tangled. Granulovacuolar degeneration involves fluid-filled cavities containing granular debris that appear within nerve cells.

According to Brookshire (1997) and Breen and Gustafson (1978), as cited by Cummings and Benson (1992), the neuritic plaques and neurofibrillary tangles occur most frequently in the temporoparietal-occipital junctions and the inferior temporal lobes. The granulovacuolar degeneration occurs most frequently in the hippocampus (part of the limbic system deep in the temporal lobe), which plays a major role in memory.

Benson and Ardila (1996) have noted that at least two varieties of Alzheimer's disease exist, each with clinical features that are clearly distinct from normal aging, and from the other disorders that cause dementia. One variety, familial Alzheimer's disease (FAD), presents a relatively early onset (before age 60), a progressive course, and many times a family history of the condition. The second variety, senile dementia of the Alzheimer's type (SDAT), also called sporadic

Alzheimer's disease, has a later age of onset, a somewhat more indolent course, and less evidence of a family history. Most clinicians group the two varieties as a single disorder called dementia of the Alzheimer's type (DAT).

Alzheimer's disease is identified by problems in language, cognition, visuospatial abilities, behavior, and motor problems in the latter stages of the condition (see chapter 1 for additional definitions). Language problems can include a *restricted vocabulary* that is limited to small talk and stereotyped cliches (Critchley, 1970), *perseveration* (Au, Obler, & Albert, 1991; Bayles, 1994; Bayles, Tomoeda, Kazniak, Stern, & Eagans, 1985; Gewirth, Shindler, & Hier, 1984), and *word-finding difficulty* (Au et al., 1991; Davis, 1993; Huff, Corkin, & Growdon, 1986).

Additional language problems can include *semantic errors* (Abeysinghe, Bayles, & Trosset, 1990; Au et al., 1991; Davis, 1993; Huff et al., 1986; Santo Pietro & Goldfarb, 1985), *naming problems* (Au et al., 1991; Bayles, 1994; Davis, 1993; Shuttleworth & Huber, 1988; Smith, Murdoch, & Chenery, 1989), *jargon* (Bayles, 1994), *circumlocution* (Au et al., 1991; Bayles, 1994; Davis, 1993), *auditory comprehension deficit* (Au et al., 1991; Davis, 1993; Eustache et al., 1995), *mutism and echolalia* (Obler & Albert, 1981), and *deficits in pragmatic language* (Bayles, 1994; Obler & Albert, 1981).

At least in the earlier stages, *syntactic* (Kempler, Curtiss, & Jackson, 1987; Rochon, Waters, & Caplan, 1994), *spelling* (Nebes & Boller, 1987; Neils, Roeltgen, & Constantinidou, 1995), and *phonologic* (Au et al., 1991; Bayles & Boone, 1982) abilities are more intact, relatively, than other language functions. A review of the nonlanguage symptoms of cortical dementia can be found in Cummings & Benson (1992).

Stages in Alzheimer's Disease

There are three stages in Alzheimer's Disease, as described in the following sections (Au et al., 1991; Bayles, 1994; Bayles, Tomoeda, & Caffrey, 1982; Benson & Ardila, 1996; Cummings & Benson, 1992).

Mild stage. During the mild stage, the patient senses a decline, becomes apologetic, and is reluctant to be tested. Frequently he or she is disoriented to time, and memory for recent events has begun to fail. The patient relies heavily on overlearned situations and stereotypical utterances, and is often unable to generate sequences of related ideas. In this stage, the patient might resemble the Wernicke's patient;

however, the Wernicke's patient cannot repeat whereas the dementia patient often can.

In this stage, the dementia patient begins to exhibit impairment semantically (slightly reduced vocabulary, word-finding difficulties, increased use of automatisms and cliches) and pragmatically (mild loss of desire to communicate, occasional disinhibitions), whereas syntactically and phonologically he or she is intact.

As an example of increased use of cliches and occasional disinhibitions, one particular patient, who was in the mild stage of dementia, was very effusive in her praise for this author as a therapist (e.g., "You're the tops," "My hat's off to you," "You're peaches and cream"). Her effusiveness was unwarranted because this author had worked with her only for a few routine but appropriate sessions. When her husband was present at our sessions, she would be very benevolent toward him. But as soon as he left, the patient accused him of seeing another woman (e.g., "He's alleycatting around," "He's acting like a wild animal"). While she related this in cliche-ridden language, her tone and manner became very aggressive. Other members of the family confirmed that the husband was faithful to his wife throughout their marriage, including this trying period.

Moderate stage. During the moderate stage, the patient has a more noticeable impairment of memory and time and place orientation, is more perseverative and nonmeaningful, and does not correct his or her own errors. In this stage, the dementia patient shows further impairment semantically (significantly reduced vocabulary, naming errors usually semantically and visually related, verbal paraphasias evident in discourse), shows some impairment syntactically (reduction in syntactic complexity and completeness), shows further impairment pragmatically (declining sensitivity to context, diminished eye contact, egocentricity), but is phonologically generally intact.

Because of difficulty with abstraction, utterances are usually concrete. Repetition begins to break down, and the patient shows circumlocutions and anomic difficulties. Eye contact begins to diminish, and there is a lot of touching of objects, indicating that the pragmatics of communication are inappropriate. Wilson, et al. (1982) found that dementia patients show a deficit in the retention of facial information. The aphasic patient would probably be adequate in this area.

Advanced stage. In the advanced stage, patients are very much disoriented to time, place, and person, and fail to recognize family and friends. They are unable to carry out the routines of life and require extensive personal care. Many times they will make spontaneous corrections of syntactic and phonologic errors, but without awareness. They have brief moments when stimuli appear to be comprehended, but for the most part they will neither comprehend nor self-correct any errors.

Their phonology is generally correct; syntax may be disturbed, but not as disturbed as the semantic aspects of language (Bayles, 1982, 1994; Bayles & Boone, 1982; Cummings & Benson, 1992). It seems that the phonologic and syntactic aspects of language remain relatively unimpaired while the semantic and pragmatic aspects are much impaired. The referential aspects of language are very disturbed but the mechanics of speech production are not, unless subcortical degeneration has taken place. In some cases, the patient could be mute except for jargon (Benson & Ardila, 1996).

In this stage, the dementia patient shows further impairment semantically (markedly reduced vocabulary, frequent unrelated misnamings, jargon common), further impairment syntactically (many inappropriate word combinations), further impairment pragmatically (nonadherence to conventional rules, poor eye contact, lack of social awareness, inability to form a purposeful intention), and some impairment phonologically (occasional phonemic paraphasias and neologisms, sometimes jargon).

As mentioned previously, a patient in the advanced stages of dementia may have verbalization that sounds very appropriate to the situation. During a speech and language diagnosis, one patient emerged from her flood of inappropriate responses by saying, "Is this necessary?" This most likely chance appropriate response was picked up by her hopeful husband, who thought that this was a sign of normal behavior. The husband was probably convinced otherwise when a few minutes later the seating arrangement shifted and brought the patient too close. She suddenly reached out, grabbed this author's tie, and held on to it for about 3 or 4 minutes. It seemed like 3 or 4 hours.

Pick's Disease

Pick's disease is yet another cortical dementia that can produce a language breakdown (Holland, McBurney, Moossy, & Reinmuth, 1985; Volin, Goldfarb, Raphael, & Weinstein, 1990). The neuropathology of this rare dementia involves the appearance of neuronal abnormalities called Pick bodies (dense globular formations) and Pick cells (enlarged neurons). In Pick's disease, personality and language impairment have an early onset, whereas the cognitive problems come later (Cummings & Benson, 1992).

Subcortical Dementia

Subcortical dementia (Cummings, 1990) is characterized by a gradual decline in cognitive abilities without any appreciable loss in associational cortical areas (language). The patient has emotional and personality changes, which are typically inertia and apathy. Memory disorders are present, and the patient has a defective ability to manipulate acquired knowledge. There is also a general slowness of information processing through the visual or auditory modality.

Benson and Ardila (1996) have noted that hypophonia is a significant problem in all subcortical dementias. The decreased voice volume usually occurs early, and unless the disease is treated the hypophonia will progress to total mutism. The speech disturbance is usually dysarthric, whereas the language disturbance tends toward the concrete and until the terminal stages is insignificant in comparison to the dysarthria.

Parkinson's disease, a degenerative disorder, is the condition that produces the majority of all subcortical dementias. About 20% to 60% of Parkinson patients will have dementia as part of their syndrome (American Psychiatric Association, 1994). Huntington's disease (a hereditary degenerative disorder); progressive supra-nuclear palsy (starts with a motor impairment and eventually a mild dementia appears); Wilson's disease, which has a juvenile type (onset in youth) and an adult type (onset between 20 and 30 years of age); olivopontocerebellar degeneration (onset between 30 and 50 years of age); and immunodeficiency virus (HIV) are other conditions that can produce subcortical dementia. Neuropathology within subcortical structures (i.e., basal ganglia, thalamus) of the brain is the cause of subcortical dementia.

Vascular Dementia

Vascular dementia (formerly called multi-infarct dementia or MID) can involve multiple infarcts (cell death caused by a loss of blood supply) in cortical, subcortical, or both areas (Cummings & Benson, 1992). Vascular dementia shows the second highest incidence and accounts for between 15% and 20% of dementia cases. Another 15% of dementia cases suffer from both Alzheimer's and vascular dementia. Vascular dementia patients will present a history that includes hypertension, heart disease, strokes, abrupt onset, focal neurologic signs, and a stepwise breakdown in their progression to dementia.

Multiple cortical infarcts can affect the anterior, middle, and/or posterior cerebral arteries, which feed such territories as the perisylvian or extrasylvian (borderzone) areas. These patients can show the symptoms of aphasia and apraxia in their progression to dementia.

Multiple subcortical infarcts are called *lacunar state* (infarcts involving the basal ganglia, thalamus, and internal capsule) or *Binswanger's disease* (infarcts involving the subcortical white matter of both hemispheres). These patients can show the symptoms of dysarthria in their progression to dementia.

Mixed Dementia

A mixed dementia would show both cortical and subcortical involvement. Individuals in this grouping would display the language abnormalities stemming from the cortical involvement, and the speech abnormalities (dysarthria, mutism, hypophonia) arising from the subcortical involvement.

According to Cummings and Benson (1992), the major causes of mixed dementia are vascular dementia (multi-infarct dementia), infectious dementia (e.g., HIV encephalopathy), toxic (e.g., drug intoxication) and metabolic (e.g., chronic anoxia), and miscellaneous dementia syndromes (e.g., posttraumatic, tumors).

Additional Sources

Additional studies and reviews of the type, speech and language disorders, and etiology of dementia can be found in Alpert, Rosen, and Welkowitz (1990); Bayles (1994); Bayles, Tomoeda, and Trosset (1992); Benson and Ardila (1996); Cummings and Benson (1992); Davis (1993); DeSanti (1997); Hier, Hagenlocker, and Shindler (1985); Marcie, Roudier,

Goldblum, and Boller (1993); Mathews, Obler, and Albert (1994); Morris (1987); and Obler and Albert (1981).

Diagnosis

Diagnostic procedures for determining the communication disorders associated with dementia can involve (a) establishing background information, (b) giving a neurologic evaluation, (c) employing tests for assessing cognition, (d) employing information about differential diagnosis, and (e) employing specific language probes.

Establishing Background Information and the Neurologic Evaluation

These procedures can be found at the beginning of the "Diagnosis" section of Chapter 3.

Tests for Assessing Cognition

The diagnosis of dementia is usually made after input from the neuropsychologist, the psychologist, the neurologist or psychiatrist, the speech–language pathologist, and other health care professionals. There are several tests that can be used for diagnosis. These include *The Global Deterioration Scale of Primary Degenerative Dementia* (GDS) (Reisberg, Ferris, DeLeon, & Crook, 1982), the *Mattis Dementia Rating Scale* (MDRS) (Mattis, 1976), and *Mini-Mental State Examination* (MMS) (Folstein, Folstein, & McHugh, 1975). For example, the MMS evaluates orientation, learning names, counting backward, spelling backward, recalling names, naming, repeating, auditory and reading comprehension, writing, and copying.

The Department of Health and Human Services has provided criteria for diagnosing Alzheimer's dementia (McKhann et al., 1984). These criteria state that if any two areas among language, memory, visuospatial orientation, and judgment are deficient along with the absence of depression, multiple infarcts, alcoholism, malnutrition, or other diseases, then a diagnosis of Alzheimer's disease is warranted.

Kempler et al. (1987) used the following to diagnose Alzheimer's dementia: (a) physical examination, (b) neurological examination, (c) neuropsychological evaluation, (d) laboratory evaluation, (e) EEG, (f) EKG, (g) chest X-ray, (h) CT scan of the head, plus cognitive dysfunction and absence of focal motor, sensory, cerebellar, and cranial nerve defects.

Ripich and Terrell (1988) employed the following criteria: (a) gradual onset and progression for at least 6 months, of sustained deterioration of memory in an alert patient, (b) impairment in at least three cognitive abilities—orientation, judgment and problem solving, functioning in community affairs, functioning in the house, functioning in personal care.

Fromm and Holland (1989) used the following criteria: (a) deficits in two or more areas of cognition, (b) a progressive worsening of memory and other cognitive functioning, (c) no disturbance of consciousness, (d) onset between the ages of 40 and 90, (e) the absence of systemic disorders or other brain diseases that could account for the progressive memory and cognitive deficits.

Differential Diagnosis

The following sections review some of the literature that relates to the differential diagnosis of dementia using language as the prime characteristic.

Dementia Versus Aphasia

Appell, Kertesz, and Fisman (1982) found that Alzheimer's patients showed symptoms that resembled those of Wernicke's and transcortical sensory aphasia more than those of Broca's or transcortical motor aphasia. Bayles et al. (1982) have noted that the dementia patient in the mild stage exhibits some semantic and pragmatic impairment; in the moderate stage, further semantic and pragmatic impairment, and some syntactic impairment; and in the advanced stage, further semantic, pragmatic, and syntactic impairment, and some phonologic impairment. In contrast, the aphasic patient at any severity level may be impaired semantically, syntactically, and phonologically (except the Wernicke's or transcortical sensory aphasic patient, whose phonology is mostly intact), but may retain pragmatic behavior that is socially appropriate.

Fromm and Holland (1989) found that Alzheimer's patients showed irrelevant, vague, and rambling responses, whereas Wernicke's aphasia patients showed perseverative, paraphasic jargon, and auditory comprehension deficit types of responses. Huff, Mack, Mahlmann, and Greenberg (1988) found that aphasic subjects have access to lexical-semantic information, but Alzheimer's patients have a loss of that information. Murdoch, Chenery, Wilks, and Boyle (1987) also found that the language deficit in the Alzheimer's patient resembled a transcortical sensory aphasia.

Nicholas, Obler, Albert, and Helm-Estabrooks (1985) found that Alzheimer's patients showed more empty phrases and conjunctions, whereas Wernicke's aphasia patients produced more neologisms, and verbal and literal paraphasias. Obler, Albert, Estabrooks, and Nicholas (1982) pointed out that more neologisms and verbal paraphasias exist in Wernicke's aphasia, whereas the Alzheimer's patient shows more logical conjunctions and comments.

Naming Ability in Dementia Versus Other Disorders

Bayles and Tomoeda (1983) and Martin and Fedio (1983) have noted a naming problem in dementia, which gets worse as the disease progresses. Benson (1979) stated that anomia in aphasic patients separates them from dementia patients. Dementia patients would have no trouble in confrontation naming but would have difficulty in producing words in categories (five fruits, five vegetables, etc.). Aphasic patients would have problems in both confrontation naming and producing words in categories. Boller et al. (1991) found that language task performance (especially naming) was the best predictor of the course of Alzheimer's patients.

Bowles, Obler, and Albert (1987) found that Alzheimer's subjects were distinguished by the number of unrelated responses in naming tasks, when compared to healthy younger and aging adults. Critchley (1970) has stated that in cases of dementia, language impairment essentially entails a poverty of language due to an inaccessibility of the speaking, writing, and reading vocabulary. The difficulty in word finding differs from the anomia of aphasic patients. The dementia patient does not necessarily show hesitancy in naming objects. Semantic errors in naming do not occur, nor do neologisms and substitutions. On the other hand, dementia patients find it difficult to name unless the real object is before them. They lapse into a sort of concrete attitude.

Horner, Heipman, Aker, Kanter, and Royall (1982) and Obler and Albert (1981) have noted that the naming errors of the dementia patient are more likely due to visual misperceptions than are the naming errors of aphasic patients, which are mostly of a semantic or phonological nature.

Overall Language Ability Within Types of Dementia Versus Other Disorders

Bayles, Boone, Tomoeda, Slauson, and Kazniak (1989) found that tasks involving memory seemed to differentiate Alzheimer's patients (poorest) from normal elderly and aphasic patients. Dick, Kean, and Sands (1989) noted that young and elderly adults showed a higher recall for internally generated words than did Alzheimer's patients. The authors attributed this to a semantic memory breakdown in the Alzheimer's subjects. Fromm, Holland, Nebes, and Oakley (1991) found that word-reading ability was sensitive to severity in the latter stages of Alzheimer's disease. Granholm and Butters (1988) noted that Alzheimer's patients were worse than Huntington's disease patients in encoding semantic relationships.

Kontiola, Laaksonen, Sulkava, and Erkin-Juntti (1990) compared the language abilities of normal elderly, Alzheimer's, and multi-infarct dementia patients. They found that the normal elderly subjects had the best language abilities, the Alzheimer's subjects showed defects in the understanding of grammatic structures, and the multi-infarct dementia subjects displayed disorders in recognition of words, naming, and repetitions. McNamara, Obler, Au, Durso, and Albert (1992) found that Parkinson's disease and Alzheimer's patients had more problems correcting output error than did normally aging subjects.

Mentis, Briggs-Whitaker, & Gramigna (1995) compared 12 Alzheimer's patients with 12 normal elderly subjects and observed significant differences between the two groups. The Alzheimer's patients were characterized by a reduced ability to change topics while preserving the discourse flow, difficulty in actively contributing to the propositional development of the topic, and a failure to maintain a topic in a clear and coherent manner. Finally, Tomoeda, Bayles, and Boone (1990) found that Alzheimer's patients performed more poorly than normal elderly subjects in auditory comprehension on tasks involving syntactic complexity.

Specific Language Probes

In testing for the communication disorders associated with dementia, Bayles (1994) has suggested using tasks that are active (nonautomatic) or generative, or that depend on logical reasoning. Active (nonautomatic) tasks call for mental and linguistic involvement. Examples are object description, story retelling, defining concepts, and explanation of sentence meaning. Generative tasks call for the conception and production of a series of related ideas or objects in a category. Examples would be naming five fruits, five vegetables, five countries, etc., or naming as many words as possible, beginning with a certain letter, within a minute's time, as in the *Word Fluency Measure* (Borkowski et al., 1967).

Logical reasoning tasks require the subject to arrive at a conclusion based on understanding similarities or differences between two or more items and the ability to use analogy. Examples are explaining the similarities or differences between a doctor and a lawyer or a farmer and a gardener, or defining proverbs (e.g., *Don't count your chickens before they hatch*) as a means of using analogy.

Questions relating to time, place, and person orientation and simple general information can be used along with the procedures described above. Where necessary, the different modalities should be used for eliciting an answer. The following questions were adapted from *Mayo Clinic Procedures for Language Evaluation* (unpublished test): What day is it? What month? What is today's date? What year? Where are you now? What city? What state? Why are you here? What are the names of significant family members? What is their relationship to you? How many children, grandchildren, etc., do you have?

In addition to these orientation questions, the clinician can ask general information questions: When do we celebrate Christmas? What is the capital of the United States? Who is the President of the United States? Before him? Who discovered America? When? How many states are there in the United States? Who was the first president of the United States? Who was president during the Civil War? Who invented Mickey Mouse and Donald Duck? What country is immediately north of the United States? Who was Helen Keller (or Mother Theresa)?

The Arizona Battery for Communication Disorders of Dementia (ABCD) (Bayles & Tomoeda, 1991) is a test for quantifying the communication disorder associated with Alzheimer's disease. The battery provides information about linguistic comprehension, linguistic expression, verbal episodic memory, mental status, and visuospatial construction. The ABCD was found to correlate highly with the *Global Deterioration Scale of Primary Degenerative Dementia* (Reisberg et al., 1982), the *Mini-Mental State Examination* (Folstein et al., 1975), and the Block Design subtest of the *Wechsler Adult Intelligence Scale* (Wechsler, 1981).

As a supplement to the tests mentioned above and to get an overall assessment of the patient's speech and language abilities, one might employ some of the assessment tools used in testing for aphasia. However, the aphasia batteries should be used in whole or in part to round out the picture, not as a definitive diagnostic tool. Horner, Dawson, Heyman, and Fish (1992) noted that it was most difficult to classify Alzheimer's patients when using the *Western Aphasia Battery* (Kertesz, 1982). A review of the tests used for evaluating dementia can be found in Bayles (1994); Cummings & Benson (1992); Davis (1993); Haynes et al. (1992); and Huber & Shuttleworth (1990).

Therapy

The first goal of therapy is to inform the patient and the caretaker(s) about the nature and the consequences of the disorder.

The dementia patient will show cognitive impairment directly correlated to the mild, moderate, and advanced stages of the condition. In cortical dementia, the language components are also affected according to the stage. In subcortical dementia, typically there is no characteristic breakdown of language, although speech can be dysarthric.

There are dementias that are reversible, which are many times caused by nutritional and metabolic conditions. Most dementias are of the progressive and irreversible type.

Because the types of dementia discussed in this chapter are of the progressive and irreversible type, spontaneous recovery and prognosis obviously play a lesser role. In some cases of Alzheimer's and Parkinson's disease, the symptoms of dementia can develop over a long period of time. These patients can remain in the mild stage for a number of years.

Regarding how dementia patients present their illness to their families, Brookshire (1997) reviewed a study by Rabins, Mace, and Lucas (1982) that questioned the families of 55 patients with irreversible dementia to ascertain what they considered the major problems in

caring for the patient. These families identified the most serious problems, in order, as physical violence, memory disturbance, catastrophic
reactions, incontinence, delusions, making accusations, hitting, and
suspiciousness.

It is generally known that speech and language therapy will not
achieve long-term improvement in the patient with dementia. However, speech and language therapy can help the patient (and the family)
to communicate maximally within the scope of his or her limited
abilities.

*The second goal of therapy is to provide the appropriate treatment
approaches and techniques.*

Efficacy of Therapy for the Communication Disorders Associated with Dementia

Although efficacy of treatment studies for communication disorders
associated with dementia are lacking, clinical reports in the literature
(see Bourgeois, 1991) indicate that therapy tasks that enhance memory;
time, place, and person orientation; word-finding abilities; functional
and daily living activities; and overall language communication between patient and family seem to be helpful for the patient. Typically,
treatment is geared toward the behavioral and speech and language
disturbances found in the mild, moderate, and advanced stages of the
disease.

Bourgeois (1991) reviewed over 100 communication treatment
studies for adults with dementia. She found that a number of treatment techniques have been successfully applied within the general
areas of changing the communication environment, controlling stimulus conditions, changing the consequences of appropriate communication, group therapy intervention, and caregivers as communication partners.

Changing the communication environment includes rearranging
furniture; adding plants, pictures, and other homey decorations; providing peers, children, and pets as conversational partners; and providing refreshments during group sessions. Controlling stimulus conditions includes external memory aids such as notebooks, calendars,
signs, labels, color codes, loudspeaker announcements, verbal prompts,
diaries, watches, cue cards, memory wallets, appointment books, 7-day

pill dispensers, reality orientation, and the enhancement of stimuli with training, or routine and repetitive exposure.

Changing the consequences of appropriate communication includes tangible reinforcers such as candy, cigarettes, and exchangeable tokens; planned ignoring; and praising correct responses. Group therapy intervention includes remotivation therapy, sensory training, resocialization therapy, reminiscence therapy, and life review therapy.

Caregivers as communication partners includes, in the mild stage, early intervention by the caregiver, education about the nature and course of the disease, and training about appropriate approaches to the patient's problem behaviors, with support group participation also recommended. In the moderate stage, caretakers provide reinforcing and stimulating communicative environments for patients.

Typically, treatment is geared toward the behavioral and communication disturbances found in the mild, moderate, and advanced stages of the disease. The therapy tasks that enhance memory; time, place, and person orientation; word-finding abilities; functional and daily living activities; and overall language communication skills can be applied in the mild stage.

In the moderate stage, the caregiver needs to be trained to be the communication facilitator, using appropriate prompts to stimulate correct responses. In the advanced stage, treatment should be caretaker-oriented, and caretakers should be taught how to provide the stimuli that will bring positive changes in the patient's behavior and communication abilities.

Managing the Memory Deficits of Persons with Mild to Moderate Dementia

Bayles and Tomoeda (1996) summarized some of the basic systems of human memory and how they are affected by the neuropathology of dementia. These authors stated that memory refers to stored knowledge and the processes for making and manipulating stored knowledge. Essential to this are the processes called activation and retrieval. Two forms of stored knowledge, or long-term memory, are delineated as *declarative* and *procedural*.

Declarative memory is fact memory, composed of semantic memory (knowledge of concepts), episodic memory (knowledge of events), and lexical memory (knowledge of words). When declarative or fact memory is activated into consciousness, it integrates with the working or active memory system. The working or active memory system activates and retrieves information and focuses attention.

Procedural memory involves the learning and implementation of motor skills (e.g., driving, playing tennis, writing). Thinking about driving would involve declarative memory, and performing the act of driving would involve procedural memory. Both declarative and procedural memory systems are typically simultaneously active and are essential parts of the working or active memory system.

During the early and middle stages, Alzheimer's disease (AD) affects working and declarative memory, but mostly spares procedural memory. The neuropathology of AD causes a proliferation of neuritic plaques, neurofibrillary tangles, and granulovacuolar degeneration in brain areas (hippocampi and basal forebrain) that are specialized for declarative and working memory. These brain areas are important in the formation of new episodic memory (events). Forgetting events which happened recently is an early symptom of AD, but as the disease advances into cortical association areas, the lexical (words) and semantic (concepts) memory systems show more deterioration.

Based on the memory systems described, Bayles & Tomoeda (1996) suggested a plan of memory therapy for AD patients that calls for linguistic manipulations that reduce the demands on episodic and working memory systems. Simplifying the form of language would include speaking in simple and short sentences, speaking slowly, and providing multi-modal cues.

Amending the content of language would include talking about the present (use of daily memory book) and not the difficult-to-remember past nor the future, talking about concrete items that the patient can see, hear, touch, and smell; using words with high frequency of occurrence; using proper nouns instead of pronouns (pronouns have difficult-to-remember antecedents); and revising and restating misunderstood language.

Modifying the use of language would include not asking questions that require the patient to search through fact (declarative) memory and recall information (e.g., instead of asking "What is your favorite TV program?" which requires a memory search, giving a choice of several TV programs, or if the disease is more severe, using a yes/no question such as "Do you like watching TV?"). AD patients often can produce meaningful language if they are engaging in an activity that they previously enjoyed. Pleasant activities that reduce fear and agitation include making a meal together, singing, crafts, simple games, and massage.

Additional Activities for the Mild Stage Patient

Listed below are some additional activities that can be employed with the dementia patient in the mild stage, and possibly in the moderate stage. The clinician should help orient the patient to time, place, and person in a concrete manner. This can be achieved through the use of visual aids such as calendars, a blackboard for large words and simple drawings, poster cards or large uncluttered pictures, daily newspapers, and photographs of family members and close friends. The clinician should also determine what functions the patient will perform in daily activities. This can include making grocery shopping lists, putting food in categories, identifying the locations and names of supermarkets, practicing money concepts coupled with simple arithmetic, and reading bus schedules (time, destinations, simple arithmetic).

1. Perform simple cooking activities (measuring with quarts, pints, pounds, ounces). Santo Pietro and Goldfarb (1995) provided specific examples for the reading of food labels (popcorn, fish fillets, and cereals), maps (city of Baltimore, shopping centers), schedules (television, recycling), food coupons (brand-name cereals), recipes (soup and stew, cookies), menus (Chinese restaurant), and price lists (airfares).

2. Set clocks and timers (seconds, minutes, hours).

3. Use the telephone for work on numbers in sequence and memory.

4. Use concrete vocabulary centered around everyday activities.

5. Participate in social and group situations to stimulate mental activity.

6. Practice orientation to family placement and relationships by using real family names. Bourgeois (1992) suggested using a naming wallet containing 30 pictures and sentences about familiar persons, places, and events that are difficult for the patient to remember.

Recently, Vanhalle, Van der Linden, Belleville, and Gilbert (1998) reported on the successful use of the Spaced Retrieval Strategy (SRS), which consists of retrieving the information to be learned after increasingly longer delays, in helping a 69-year-old Alzheimer's patient to recall names.

The third goal of therapy is to encourage the patient and the caretaker(s) to continue the rehabilitative process outside of the clinical setting.

Rehabilitation at Home

Bayles et al. (1982) and Bourgeois (1991) pointed out that the family and caretakers can make many modifications in the way they communicate with the patient, to facilitate the comprehension and retention of information. Rate of speech, level of syntactic complexity, and the mode of linguistic input may all affect the patient's comprehension. Verbal analogies, fragmented discourse, humor, sarcasm, use of indefinite referents, conversation involving more than two individuals, and open-ended questions are the types of language that are hardest for the dementia patient. Providing conversational partners (peers, children, etc.) and rewarding appropriate communication with tangible reinforcers (food, etc.) will also facilitate communication.

In addition, those authors and *Mayo Clinic Health Letter* "Dementia," (1995) suggested counseling the family to do the following

1. Maintain a simple routine.

2. Maintain a constant environment (dressing, eating, etc.).

3. Be consistent.

4. Minimize distractions.

5. Keep your loved one involved.

6. Reassign household chores.

7. Join support groups for families and/or patient.

8. Give yourself a break for reenergizing.

9. Keep some hobbies that renew your mental or physical strength.

10. Expect the patient to deny the problem.

11. Expect the affected individual to become anxious.

12. Simplify verbal interactions.

13. Expect a change in the patient's condition if there is a major change in lifestyle.

14. Avoid arguing with the affected individual.

15. Dispense the patient's medication and make sure the patient eats and exercises properly.

16. Have the patient wear an identification bracelet.

17. Put sensors under the rug in case the patient roams at inappropriate times.

18. Install complicated door locks.

Bayles and Tomoeda (1996) also suggested a plan of memory therapy for AD patients that calls for nonlinguistic manipulations that reduce the demand on episodic memory (events) and capitalize on procedural (motor activity) and recognition memory.

AD patients quite often have difficulty in feeding themselves. This functional motor skill can be helped by the following:

1. feeding the patient in the same place

2. positioning the food so that it can be seen

3. eliminating distractions

4. placing eating utensil in patient's hand

5. providing a model of the actual eating act

6. pairing touch with the start of feeding

7. pacing feeding so that time between bites is about the same

8. using social reinforcements for self-feeding (e.g., verbal compliments, touching)

9. providing beverages routinely

10. using finger food where possible

Orange, Lubinski, and Higginbotham (1996) examined the conversational repair (the efforts of conversational partners to correct and resolve misunderstandings or mishearing) of 6 normal elderly adults, 5 subjects with early stage dementia of the Alzheimer's type (EDAT), and 5 subjects with middle stage DAT (MDAT), with a family member who acted as a conversational partner. The percentage of conversation involved in repair was significantly higher for MDAT versus control and EDAT subjects. Despite the increase of conversational troubles with DAT onset and progression, the difficulties were repaired successfully a majority of the time. These findings have implications for developing caregiver communication enhancement strategies that are specific to the clinical stage of DAT. The authors provided examples of the trouble sources, repair initiators, repairs, and resolutions of conversational repair.

Recently, Orange and Colton-Hudson (1998) reported on how a communication education and training program (a) helped the spouse in coping with her husband's illness (dementia of the Alzheimer's type, DAT), (b) produced fewer instances of communication breakdown between the two, (c) produced greater use of efficient techniques to signal and repair communication problems, (d) showed a decrease in negative emotional responses to challenging behaviors, and (e) produced a positive response to the implementation and completion of the program.

Rehabilitation in a Facility

Long-term care facilities that provide the consistent routines, familiar environments, and appropriate cultural markers (art, music, dress, language, food, and surrounding decor) that were part of the patients' premorbid lives, can greatly enhance the patients' ability to maintain skills. There is a trend toward designing nurturing environments in long-term care facilities for dementia patients.

Recently, Johnson and Bourgeois (1998) reported on how a respite program helped a 90-year-old dementia patient increase her initiation of conversational topics, and how the patient's daughter received temporary relief from caregiving and specific instructions for helping her mother at home. The patient's swallowing and auditory acuity problems were also addressed.

Additional Memory Helpers

Although the following memory guidelines (Hearst Business Communications, Inc.) are geared for the normally aging person, they can be adapted quite easily for use with a dementia patient in the mild stage.

1. Take time to remember. Train yourself to become more aware by pausing before you go anywhere or say anything. Take a deep breath, clear your throat, relax.

2. Write notes and lists. Whenever you think of something you have to do, try to do it right away. If you can't get to the task, write it down. This is especially useful when there is too much to do and too little time.

3. Establish routines. Set up habits such as storing keys, your pocketbook, and/or your wallet in a certain place each time you put them down.

4. Don't become distracted. Any type of distraction will hinder your ability to recall information. If you tend to do several things at the same time, choose priorities and try to do one thing after the other.

5. Keep mentally active. Play games, join a study group, take a class to keep your mind alert. For example, start doing crossword puzzles, anagrams, or play Monopoly.

6. Rehearse information. Before you go to a party or class reunion, review the names of people you will be seeing and visualize them in the context in which you know them.

7. Create a mental picture. "Seeing" something can help you recall a name or other information. For example, develop a mental picture of a store when trying to recall the name of the business.

8. Keep physically active. Exercise seems to have a positive effect on mental abilities; even a little physical activity can help mental awareness.

9. Beware of fatigue. When tired or under stress, pay even more attention to normal daily tasks. If at all possible, postpone doing tasks until fully rested.

10. Don't doubt yourself. Most important, don't question your ability. By doubting yourself, you can make a situation worse by exaggerating every memory lapse.

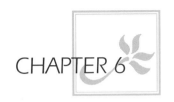

CHAPTER 6

Communication Disorders Associated with Traumatic Brain Injury

Definition and Etiology

Traumatic brain injury (TBI) occurs when a swiftly moving object hits the head (e.g., bullet wounds), or when the moving head strikes a stationary object (e.g., falls). Coelho (1997) noted that the damage following TBI is the result of primary and secondary damage, along with physiologic changes that can affect brain function. Primary damage is caused by the actual impact to the brain. Secondary damage is a consequence of such factors as infection, hypoxia, edema, elevated intracranial pressure, infarction, and hematomas. Physiologic changes can result from a number of metabolic disturbances such as hyperthermia, electrolyte imbalances, and damage to the hypothalamus or pituitary gland.

Open head injury (or penetrating brain injury) is where the skull is fractured or perforated, and the meninges are torn or lacerated. In open head injuries, *primary damage* usually occurs along the path of the penetrating object (shrapnel, stones, bullets, blunt or sharp instruments). *Secondary damage* can result from the effects of swelling, bleeding, infections, increased intracranial pressure, and scarring.

Closed head injury (or nonpenetrating brain injury) is where the meninges (three layers of tissue that cover the brain) remain intact.

Trauma at the point of impact is known as coup. Injuries to the brain on the opposite side from the point of impact are known as contrecoup. In closed head injuries, *primary damage* usually occurs because the brain is involved in high levels of acceleration and deceleration (e.g., automobile and motorcycle accidents, falls). The rapid twisting and rotation of the brain can result in a shearing, stretching, or tearing of nerve fibers and is identified as diffuse axonal injury. As mentioned previously, *secondary damage* can occur as a result of such factors as infection, hypoxia (lack of oxygen), edema (swelling), elevation of intracranial pressure, infarction (cell death due to lack of oxygen in the brain), and hematomas (accumulation of blood from a hemorrhage).

Deep coma is a state of profound unconsciousness where the person cannot be aroused and makes no response to external stimuli (e.g., pain, sound, touch, smell). The lightest stages of coma are where the person responds to external stimuli but in a general and nonspecific manner (e.g., whole body or nonspecific motor movements). Coma can occur through interference with the reticular system of the brain, which is responsible for attention and alertness. Coma is more prevalent in closed head injury than in open head injury because of the widespread damage caused by diffuse axonal injury.

Traumatic brain injury (Adamovich, 1992; Coelho, 1997; Netsell & Lefkowitz, 1992; Sarno, Buonaguro, & Levita, 1986) can also cause aphasia, the communication disorders associated with right hemisphere damage, dysarthria, and apraxia of speech, all of which are discussed elsewhere in this book. The symptoms described in the next section typically result from diffuse brain damage.

Symptoms

The communication disorder discussed here is a condition that can fit into the category labeled by ASHA (1991) as cognitive-communicative disorders. Adamovich (1992), Brookshire (1997), Coelho (1997), Davis (1993), Hartley (1994), and Ylvisaker and Szekeres (1994) have elaborated on the origin of this communication breakdown. The factors to consider are cognitive, executive, linguistic, and behavioral functioning.

Cognitive Functioning

Cognitive functioning involves orientation, arousal, attention, speed of processing, memory (see Chapter 5 for further discussion of memory), abstract reasoning, and visuospatial perception (see Chapter 1 for definitions). Because attention and memory problems are so prevalent in the TBI patient, an expanded description is presented in the following paragraphs.

Mateer (1996) reviewed the various models of attention that can be used to assess and treat disorders of the attentional system such as TBI. One of them is the clinical model of attention (Sohlberg & Mateer, 1989). The model is hierarchical, with each level viewed as more complex and requiring effective functioning at the previous level. Components of the model are as follows:

1. *Focused attention.* This is the ability to respond discretely to specific visual, auditory, or tactile stimuli (e.g., looking at a glass globe in which snow or confetti moves when the globe is turned upside down). This level does not imply purposefulness of response.

2. *Sustained attention.* This is the ability to maintain a consistent behavioral response during continuous and repetitive activity (e.g., matching playing cards correctly according to number, color, or suit). This level incorporates concepts of vigilance.

3. *Selective attention.* This is the ability to maintain a behavioral or cognitive set in the face of distracting or competing stimuli (e.g., paying attention to the clinician even though a television is playing or other people are in the background). This level incorporates the concept of "freedom from distractibility."

4. *Alternating attention.* This is the capacity for mental flexibility that allows one to shift his or her focus of attention and move between tasks that have different cognitive requirements or require different behavior responses (e.g., attending correctly to the clinician, then properly responding to a phone call or visitor who interrupts, and then correctly resuming with the clinician). This level controls which information will be selectively attended to, and incorporates the concept of shifting an established set easily.

5. *Divided attention.* This is the ability to respond simultaneously to multiple tasks or multiple task demands (e.g., attending correctly to the clinician, while keeping track of a child in the same room). At this level,

two or more behavioral responses may be required, or two or more kinds of stimuli may need to be monitored.

Memory is an essential aspect of cognitive functioning. TBI patients are quite susceptible to pretraumatic and posttraumatic amnesia.

Pretraumatic amnesia is the loss of memory for events occurring before the trauma. Often the patient cannot remember the minutes, hours, or even days before the injury. The memory loss can last for up to a year, sometimes longer. As the patient begins to recover, the memory loss preceding the trauma gets shorter in terms of the time period mentioned. Pretraumatic amnesia may be caused by problems with the retrieval processes.

Posttraumatic amnesia refers to the loss of memory for events occurring after the trauma. The memory loss can last for several minutes, hours, days, months, and in some cases, years. As the patient begins to recover, memory for day-to-day events slowly becomes better. Posttraumatic amnesia is the more serious problem of the two because it involves everyday activities and appears to be a problem involving storage of memory processes.

Executive Functioning

Executive functioning includes goal setting, awareness of self, initiation of goal-directed behavior, sequencing, planning, organizing, monitoring and controlling behavior, problem solving, and self-evaluation. Some examples of executive functioning would be planning one's daily activities (e.g., getting dressed); how one gets to the doctor; the steps used in preparing foods; arranging items from large to small or vice versa; arranging items from most to least important; putting theme cards in a logical sequence (e.g., supermarket shopping from start to finish; taking a cab from beginning to end of destination); looking at the success or failure in performing a particular task and knowing why it succeeded or failed and the steps needed to rectify the failure; and so forth. (See Chapter 5 for additional comments on executive dysfunction.)

Linguistic Functioning

A linguistic functioning problem can occur because of a lesion in a language area of the brain; this would be called aphasia. In aphasia, com-

munication is impaired because the components of language (phonologic, morphologic, syntactic, and semantic) are directly interfered with.

Linguistic functioning problems also can be caused by a lesion or
lesions in parts of the brain that control cognitive and executive functioning and behavior; this would be called a cognitive-communicative
disorder. In a cognitive-communicative disorder, communication is
impaired because the components of cognition (orientation, arousal,
attention, speed of processing, memory, abstract reasoning, and visuospatial perception), executive functioning, and behavior are directly interfered with, and this in turn indirectly interferes with language.
For example, an aphasic patient will have an auditory comprehension
problem due to a lesion in Wernicke's or other areas, and he will respond
erroneously because he didn't understand the instruction (e.g., "Point to
the window"). A cognitive-communicative disorder patient will have an
auditory comprehension problem and give an erroneous response
because from among several possibilities, her attention span for the auditory stimulus (e.g., "Point to the window") was limited or wandering.

Darley (1982), Halpern, Darley, and Brown (1973), and Wertz (1985)
have called this condition the language of confusion where, because of
deficits in cognition, the patient usually manifests an inability to follow
directions, bizarre and irrelevant responses (see Drummond, 1986),
unawareness of the inappropriateness of his or her responses, and confabulations (a fictitious story reported through oral and/or written
expression). Dalla Barba (1993) has reviewed the different patterns of
confabulation and noted that confabulation is different from lying,
where there is intention to deceive. (See Chapter 4 for additional discussion of confabulation).

Geschwind (1967) described the syndrome of "nonaphasic misnaming," which typically occurs in disorders that diffusely involve the
nervous system, especially when the disturbance comes on fairly
rapidly. Characteristically the errors tend to "propagate." Thus the
patient, if asked where he or she is, may say, "in a bus," and may continue by identifying the examiner as the bus driver, those around her as
passengers, and her bed as one being used by the driver for resting.

It is usually obvious, once a sequence of questions is asked, that
ordinary aphasic misnaming is readily ruled out. In aphasic misnaming
there is no tendency to propagation, although perseveration (e.g., repetition of the same incorrect word) occurs frequently. The connected or
propagated character of the errors may show up particularly in relation

to the hospital and the patient's illness. The patient may call the hospital a "hotel," the doctors "bellboys," and the nurses "chambermaids," and will not accept correction.

Stengel (1964) stated that people in confusional states, when called upon to name objects, do not respond in the same way as aphasics, who say, "I know what it is, but I can't find the word." Confused patients boldly and sometimes recklessly improvise and produce words on the spur of the moment. These words may show effects of perseveration, slang, and other associations.

Weinstein, Lyerly, Cole, and Ozer (1966) used the term "jargon aphasia" to describe subjects who had bilateral brain involvement and showed confabulation, particularly about the onset of the illness as the reason for coming to the hospital; disorientation for place and time; unawareness of errors; and lack of any catastrophic response.

From the studies cited, it is obvious that among the language skills, the factor of impairment of relevance is a key differentiating point. In working with a TBI patient, this author found the following to be typical examples of irrelevant responses: "A measure of violence" was given as the definition for *bargain*. "Should watch out for mail boxes, should watch out for people, should watch out for papers" was a response to the question, "What three things should every good citizen do?" In response to this same question, another TBI patient said, "Have your tires checked, know a good auto shop, buy a Ford, and go to Sears."

Davis (1993), Hartley (1994), and Ylvisaker and Szekeres (1994) reviewed a number of studies about the language deficits that occur after TBI. These studies have revealed that (a) TBI can produce deficits in all four modalities and at all levels of severity, as does aphasia; (b) there are fewer cases of aphasia after TBI in acute care facilities than there are in rehabilitation centers; (c) the predominant kind of aphasia after TBI is fluent and anomic; (d) language therapy for aphasia caused by TBI is generally the same as for aphasia caused by CVA.

Behavioral Functioning

Behavioral functioning impairment can manifest itself as irritability and aggression, anxiety, depression, decreased initiation, disinhibition, and social inappropriateness. (See Treatment for Mild Impairment in this chapter.)

Diagnosis

Diagnostic procedures for determining the communication disorders associated with traumatic brain injury can involve (a) establishing background information, (b) giving a neurologic evaluation, (c) employing tests for assessing cognition and language, and (d) employing information about differential diagnosis.

Establishing Background Information and the Neurologic Evaluation

These procedures can be found at the beginning of the "Diagnosis" section of Chapter 3.

Tests for Assessing Cognition and Language

Depending upon which stage of recovery the TBI patient is in, different diagnostic procedures can be used. If the patient is severely impaired, *The Glasgow Coma Scale* (Jennett & Teasdale, 1981) evaluates eye opening abilities, motor responses, and verbal responses. Eye opening items include: (a) opens eyes spontaneously (best score), (b) opens eyes to verbal command, (c) opens eyes in response to pain, and (d) no response (worst score). Motor response items include: (a) obeys verbal commands (best score), (b) attempts to pull examiner's hand away during painful stimulation, (c) moves limb away from painful stimulus, (d) flexes body in response to pain, (e) extends limbs, becomes rigid in response to pain, and (f) no response (worst score). Verbal response items include: (a) converses and is oriented (best score), (b) converses but is disoriented, (c) utters intelligible words but does not make sense, (d) produces unintelligible sounds, and (e) no response (worst score).

Another instrument is *The Rancho Los Amigos Scale of Cognitive Levels* (Hagen, 1984), which evaluates the patient's cognitive and behavioral course of recovery. The test measures the patient's responses to stimuli that range from Level I—No Response (no response to pain, touch, sound, or sight) to Level VIII—Purposeful and Appropriate (responds appropriately in most situations, can generalize new learning across situations, does not require daily supervision, may have poor tolerance for stress and may exhibit some abstract reasoning disabilities).

Many TBI patients suffer from posttraumatic amnesia. *The Galveston Orientation and Amnesia Test* (GOAT) (Levin, O'Donnell, & Grossman, 1979) can be used to assess the patient's memory, amnesia, and orientation. The memory portion evaluates short-term memory for words, the alphabet, and counting backward. The amnesia portion asks the patient to tell his or her name, place of birth, age, and where he or she lives. The orientation portion checks the patient's knowledge of time (year, month, day, hour) and place (present location).

Currently, there are two tests that can evaluate the TBI patient's cognitive and linguistic abilities. One is the *Brief Test of Head Injury* (BTHI) (Helm-Estabrooks & Hotz, 1990), which is designed to assess orientation and attention, following commands, linguistic organization, reading comprehension, naming, memory, and visuospatial skills. Items are scored by type of response (linguistic, gestural), and communicative quality of the response. The other is *The Scales of Cognitive Ability for Traumatic Brain Injury* (SCATBI) (Adamovich & Henderson, 1992), which is constructed to evaluate perception/discrimination, orientation, organization, recall, and reasoning.

Although most batteries that assess cognition are conceived by individuals in other professions, the two preceding tests were designed by speech–language pathologists. It is quite important to know not only for assessment, but for the treatment that follows whether the problem in communication is due to a direct language impairment (aphasia) or an indirect language problem due to an impairment in cognition that impedes communication in a certain way.

Finally, *The Ross Information Processing Assessment* (RIPA–2) (Ross-Swain, 1996) can be used to test communicative and cognitive functioning (see Chapter 4 for additional description), and *The Discourse Comprehension Test* (Brookshire and Nicholas, 1997) assesses both listening and reading comprehension (see Chapter 3, "Diagnosis").

Differential Diagnosis

The findings of the following studies can be used to aid in the language diagnosis. The language findings of the study by Halpern et al. (1973) indicated that the group with confused language was differentiated from the other groups (aphasia, generalized intellectual impairment,

language of confusion

and apraxia of speech) by impairment in reading comprehension, writing words to dictation, and relevance.

Groher (1977) studied the memory and language skills of 14 patients who had suffered closed head trauma. He noted that initially his subjects manifested both aphasic (a reduced capacity to interpret and formulate language symbols) and confused language skills (faulty short-term memory, mistaken reasoning, inappropriate behavior, poor understanding of the environment, and disorientation). After a period of 1 month, both language and memory skills improved significantly. Continued improvement was made after 1 month and up to 4 months in both language and memory abilities, although deficits were still present in both areas at 4 months.

Comparing a single patient with the language of confusion with 10 aphasic patients, Mills and Drummond (1980) found that naming ability could be used as a discriminating factor between the two disorders. The factors of error rate and response time in naming tasks were more variable in the patient with the language of confusion than in the aphasic patients. The greatest error rate and the longest response time took place in the early stages of recovery in the patient with confused language. In the latter stages of recovery, error rate and response time were close to normal. The aphasic patients were consistent throughout this time period. A greater percentage of semantically unrelated responses was found in the patient with confused language than in the aphasia group.

In another study of a single patient with the language of confusion, Drummond (1984) noted that a monologue context ("Tell me how you would fry an egg") was more effective for observing linguistic irrelevancy than picture description. The monologue context provides a topic and requires the speaker to introduce different referents, expand on each of these referents, and then arrange them in a temporal hierarchy utilizing the past, present, and future. She also found that total utterance and impaired topic-focus organization were probably the most valid variables for describing linguistic irrelevancy. Both of these factors diminish progressively with physiological recovery.

Ehrlich (1988) found that in picture description tasks, adults with head injury were more verbose and slower than normal subject in imparting information. Liles, Coelho, Duffy, and Zalagens (1989) observed that adults with closed head injury were differentiated from normal subjects by story generation and story retelling tasks. Tompkins et al. (1990) found that injury severity, and existence and severity of previous psychological, physical, or cognitive disorders were the best predictors of recovery for adults with closed head injury. In children with closed head injury, parental marital status was the best predictor.

Gruen, Frankle, and Schwartz (1990) measured the word fluency generation tasks (animal naming and single-letter based word generation) of 218 closed head injury subjects, and noted significant differences in response quality and quantity relative to normal subjects. Peach (1992) found that perceptual functioning, general language abilities, and mental efficiency were the major factors underlying neuropsychological test performance in chronic severe TBI.

Campbell and Dollaghan (1990, 1995) conducted two studies to examine the speaking rate following TBI in 9 children and adolescents. Study I (1990) showed that the average speaking rate of the group with TBI was slower than that of the age-matched control subjects. Study II (1995) showed that articulatory speed and linguistic processing speed may contribute independently to slowed speaking rates more than 1 year after TBI.

Therapy

The first goal of therapy is to inform the patient and the caretaker(s) about the nature and the consequences of the disorder.

The TBI patient will show cognitive impairment directly related to the mild (or late), moderate (or middle), and severe (or early) stages of the condition. The language components are affected according to the stage of the disorder.

Ylvisaker and Szekeres (1994) noted the stages of recovery for the closed head injury (CHI) patient, which falls under the heading of TBI. These stages are based on the *Rancho Los Amigos Scale of Cognitive Levels* (Hagen, 1984), which is an eight-stage recovery scale. The *early stage (severe impairment)* starts with the first generalized responses to the environment (inconsistent responses to pain, touch, sound, or sight) and ends with stimulus-specific responses (e.g., visual tracking, localizing to sound), recognition of some common objects, and comprehension of some simple commands. The *middle stage (moderate impairment)* starts with heightened alertness and increased activity, along with confusion and agitation, and ends with improved orientation and behavior that is generally goal-directed, and can consistently follow simple directions. The *late stage (mild impairment)* starts with adequate orientation (although insight, judgment, and problem solving may be poor) and performance of daily routine tasks in a highly familiar environment (usually done in an automatic, robot-like manner) and ends with the patient's responding appropriately in most situations and generalizing new learning across most situations (some abstract reasoning abilities may still be impaired). Patients do not require daily supervision but may have poor tolerance for stress.

The second goal of therapy is to provide the appropriate treatment approaches and techniques.

Efficacy of Therapy for the Communication Disorders Associated with Traumatic Brain Injury

Recently, Coelho, DeRuyter, and Stein (1996) reviewed several treatment efficacy studies of cognitive rehabilitation. In their review, they found that there are a number of treatment techniques that have been successfully applied to deficits of attention, memory, and executive function in various TBI patients. Patients with more severe cognitive-communicative deficits can receive treatment directed toward the development of compensatory strategies, such as the use of memory aids (e.g., appointment book, alarm watch, or a detailed daily schedule).

For patients with profound deficits, the treatment may best be focused on environmental modifications or the arrangement of permanent support systems (e.g., training caretakers to prompt the patient during daily living activities). Single-subject, multiple baseline designs are well suited for studying the efficacy of these treatment approaches to cognitive rehabilitation. Social skills retraining, timing of treatment during recovery, treatment location and its effectiveness (e.g., hospital, home, school, work), and the benefits of early intervention were also stressed.

Coelho et al. (1996) noted that functional gains were realized in receptive and expressive language, speech production, reading, writing, and cognition for TBI patients receiving speech–language treatment. Inpatients receiving cognitive rehabilitation returned to productive living at the same rate as a less severely impaired group who had not received treatment. When patients with similar severity were compared, those who had received cognitive rehabilitation had better average cost outcomes than those not receiving rehabilitation services.

Cognitive Rehabilitation

Coelho (1997) stated that the treatment of cognitive-communicative disorders that arises from TBI is known as cognitive rehabilitation. Cognitive rehabilitation embodies a treatment program directed at raising functional abilities in everyday activities. This is done primarily by improving the patient's ability to process and interpret incoming information. The two approaches to cognitive rehabilitation are restorative and compensatory.

The restorative approach is based on neuronal growth through repetitive exercises and drilling of neuronal circuits. The compensatory approach is based on circumventing the impaired functions. Usually, the restorative approach is used first, and if that doesn't work, the compensatory approach is implemented. After awhile, these approaches can be used simultaneously in therapy to achieve functional abilities in everyday life.

Treatment for Severe Impairment (Early Stage)

Because of problems primarily in arousal, attention, orientation, and pretraumatic and posttraumatic amnesia, communicative functioning can be very limited. Treatment is geared on a basic functional level, toward stimulating those problem areas. For early stage or slow-to-recover patients, Ansell (1991) suggested the following (with some adaptation) sensory stimulation examples:

1. Present visual stimuli (e.g., a glass globe with "snow" or confetti that moves when the globe is turned upside down, or a colorful pinwheel) to engage the patient's attention and facilitate visual tracking.

2. Give orientation information to patients, including greeting them by name; identifying the clinician by name and title;

and telling patient the day, date, name of facility in which the patient resides, the length of time the patient has been there, and the reason for his or her placement at the facility.

3. Present multi-sensory stimulation to facilitate auditory comprehension (e.g., put a soft ball in the patient's hand and aid in squeezing the ball while saying "Squeeze the ball").

4. Present tactile/gustatory stimulation to the lips via flavored popsicles, to facilitate purposeful oral movement and awareness/recognition of flavors and temperature. Olfactory stimuli (e.g., extracts, perfumes, colognes, spices, soaps, vinegar) and additional gustatory stimuli (e.g., extracts, lemon, vinegar) have also been recommended to see if the patient consistently reacts and to assess the nature of that reaction.

If the patient is progressing in his or her recovery, the clinician can begin the early application of environmental modification. Ylvisaker and Szekeres (1994) suggested some forms of environmental modification. These activities include developing and practicing routines to structure the patient's day (e.g., time to get up, shower, dress, eat breakfast, therapy appointments). Visual cues such as pictures of personnel, calendars, date books, signs, and posters of upcoming events will help the patient acquire and maintain control of his or her environment.

Treatment for Moderate Impairment (Middle Stage)

Treatment in this stage consists of continuing and elaborating on environmental modification and ameliorating the patient's cognitive impairment. Adamovich (1992) suggested the following activities for bolstering cognition. They are presented here with some adaptation.

1. *Perception.* Visual and auditory perceptual tasks involve tracking and scanning; perception of sounds, words, and objects (e.g., use large print, use finger or card to maintain place, place items in best visual field, request repetition through auditory mode, request slowing down through auditory mode, request breakdown of smaller units of infor-

mation through auditory mode); tracing or copying; following simple commands; and naming objects.

2. *Discrimination.* Activities begin with the visual discrimination of colors, shapes, and sizes followed by the discrimination of pictures, words, sentences, and situations (e.g., matching of colors; classifying from light to dark; classifying round or long shapes; classifying small to large; putting words, sentences, and situations into categories, themes, function) and seeing how many stimulus items can be handled by the patient at once. This is progression from one to two, three, four, and more items at the same time.

3. *Organization.* Organizational skills include the categorization or grouping of items by physical attributes, meaningful units, function, likenesses, and differences (e.g., grouping objects according to round or long shapes, or small or large items; grouping words according to fruits or vegetables, or cities). Closure activities include the identification of missing elements of pictures, letters, words, sentences, stories, conversations, and situations. Sequencing activities include the sequencing of visual information (e.g., smallest to largest, lightest to darkest); sequencing of letters (e.g., from *A* to *Z*), words, and sentences (e.g., putting parts of a letter—date, *Dear Sir,* body of letter, *Sincerely Yours,* signature, and postscript—in their proper order); and sequencing functional activities (e.g., taking a shower, making coffee, frying an egg, shopping).

4. *Recall/Memory.* Treatment of memory disturbances includes internal retrieval strategies and external memory aids. Internal strategies include rehearsal, associations, and mnemonic devices. External memory aids include calendars, appointment books, note pads, daily logs/diaries, memo pads, lists, structured routines, reminder alarms, tape recorders, and watch alarms. For additional items that improve the ability to recall information, see Chapter 5.

5. *Reasoning/Problem Solving.* Several types of reasoning should be addressed, beginning with the most concrete (e.g., Will your car fit into the parking space?) and extending to more abstract reasoning (e.g., You forgot where you parked your car at a large shopping mall; figure out where it is by thinking through which mall entrance you came into, which store you shopped at first, which section of the department store you entered first, etc.). Additional activities can include simple arithmetic problems, simple maze designs, analogies, same and different aspects (e.g., doctor–lawyer), etc.

Treatment for Mild Impairment (Late Stage)

Executive and Behavior Problems

Due to frontal lobe damage, the TBI patient will quite often have problems in executive function and behavior. Lezak (1982) described *executive functioning* as the ability to think about goals (e.g., a graduate student thinks about a topic for a term paper as part of a course requirement which will lead to a graduate degree), develop a plan (e.g., the same graduate student thinks about whether the format of the paper should be an experimental design, a case study, a review and analysis of the literature, etc., and whether symptoms, etiology, diagnosis, or therapy or any combination of these areas will be covered), and successfully execute the plan (e.g., the same graduate student goes to the library, tests subjects if applicable, gathers and analyzes data, types it up, and completes it in time to hand in to the instructor).

Jacobs (1992) noted that the *behavioral problems* of the TBI patient include anxiety, depression, withdrawal, aggressive behavior, temperament, decreased initiation, poor self-control, and attention seeking. These behavior problems can be caused directly by a lesion in particular areas of the brain that govern behavior (e.g., frontal and temporal lobes), or indirectly by a lesion in areas that govern cognition (e.g., attention, perception, memory, orientation), an impairment that can produce aberrant behavior when the patient tries to cope.

Behavior problems can also occur when the patient is trying to cope with associated injuries (e.g., amputation of limbs), or because of environmental factors that cause the patient to react or cope erratically (e.g., adjusting to a noisy or stuffy room, getting used to personnel). Many times, the behavior problems decrease as the patient regains cognitive abilities, executive function, and language abilities, and adjusts to the environment. Some patients may need additional treatment (e.g., counseling, medication).

Problems in executive function and behavior may have been present in the first two stages of recovery, but become most apparent in the last stage. It is during this stage that the TBI patient plans to re-enter society. Taking on and completing everyday activities (e.g., dressing, eating breakfast, preparing to go to school or work) are interwoven with a good deal of social interaction which, of course, involves the use of language.

Executive Function Deficits

As suggested by Brookshire (1997), and Ylvisaker and Szekeres (1994), treatment for executive function problems might include the following:

1. Break complex and demanding tasks into smaller segments.

2. Ask others to write down complex instructions and schedules.

3. Establish consistent routines and regular schedules for daily activities.

4. Get help from family members, friends, and associates in how to successfully ease the patient into daily life activities.

5. Keep possessions in designated places.

6. Organize the work space and set aside specific times for work at difficult tasks (i.e., when patient is rested and alert).

7. Set time limits (using alarms, timers) for working at difficult tasks.

8. Use a written daily schedule of events and appointments, with a place to check them off when completed.

9. Use an alarm watch or timer to signal appointments or other scheduled duties or events.

10. Use a daily log in which the day's activities can be recorded by the patient and/or others.

11. Place signs or notes in strategic locations as reminders for certain activities (e.g., Do you have your keys?).

Recently, Cazzato (1998) reported on the use of functionally based rehabilitation with a mild TBI patient. Complex attention skills, organizational activities, and memory strategies were worked on in the clinical setting and then in the actual work setting (the patient's home office). The patient's job required a great deal of travel and phone contact, and the need to structure and organize time and schedules. Referring to spreadsheets on the computer, making phone calls, collecting mailings, and sending or receiving faxes, all occurring in rapid succession or simultaneously, were at first simulated in the clinic. These activities were then shifted into the patient's home office, where the functional setting allowed for treatment gains to be generalized more effectively than in the clinical setting.

Language and Discourse Problems

Hartley (1994) noted that the area of language most likely affected during social interaction is discourse. Social interaction requires the blending of cognitive, social–behavioral, executive, and language skills. The discourse of TBI patients has been described as tangential, confused, and inappropriate in content and length. Hartley reviewed several studies dealing with narrative discourse after TBI; problems included decreased use of cohesive ties, decreased amount of information conveyed, use of ambiguous pronouns, slowed rate of production, excessive dysfluencies, and use of shorter sentences.

Nicholas and Brookshire (1995a) reviewed several studies and concluded that impaired listening comprehension is a frequent problem with TBI. Using an earlier version of their *Discourse Comprehension Test* (see Chapter 3), they found that in the comprehension of spoken narrative discourse, 20 TBI subjects had more correct responses when questions assessed main ideas than when they assessed details, and more correct responses when questions assessed stated information than when they assessed implied information. In addition, stated information had stronger effects on their comprehension of details than on their comprehension of main ideas.

Some treatment suggestions by Brookshire (1997) and Ylvisaker and Szekeres (1994) for problems in language, specifically discourse, include the following:

1. Use scripts (e.g., going to a restaurant, shopping in the supermarket) to generate real or imagined descriptions of experiences.

2. Note topic of any conversation. *What are we talking about right now?*

3. Self-examine regarding the main point.

4. Alert others before shifting topics.

5. Rehearse important comments and self-examine.

6. Ask for clarification or repetition when confused about what others are saying.

7. Watch others for feedback as to whether your comments are clear.

8. Watch facial expression of listener or ask about clarity of your remarks.

9. Practice retelling a story (e.g., view a picture story and then express it verbally).

10. Practice generating a story (e.g., view a single action picture and create a narrative for it).

The third goal of therapy is to encourage the patient and the caretaker(s) to continue the rehabilitative process outside of the clinical setting.

Treatment for Attention Deficit

Mateer (1996) suggested several attention compensation techniques for use with TBI patients. These techniques to enhance concentration include the following:

1. Reduce distractions (e.g., turn off radio, TV, or loud machinery, close curtains, close eyes, use earplugs).

2. Avoid crowds (e.g., shop and drive during off-hours in small stores and streets, visit with people in small numbers, if a crowd is unavoidable take someone who can assist or act as a guide if necessary).

3. Watch out for fatigue (e.g., take frequent breaks when starting to get overwhelmed or nearing information overload).

4. Avoid interruptions (e.g., unplug phone or use answering machine, use a "Do Not Disturb" sign, ask others not to interrupt, do only one thing at a time).

5. Get enough sleep and exercise (e.g., naps and physical exercise help both sleep and attention).

6. Ask for help (e.g., tell trusted ones about your problems and ask for assistance, if needed, for items mentioned above).

Treatment for Confabulations

Recently, Sohlberg and Ehlhardt (1998) reported on assisting a caregiver in data collection and analysis of the confabulations uttered by a patient who also exhibited memory loss and personality change. The caregiver was provided with some education about the nature of confabulations (e.g., accompany memory loss, no intent to deceive, due to brain damage).

The hope was that the caretaker (the mental health counselor) and the staff would develop strategies for managing and decreasing the confabulations, which indeed they did. The most interesting result was that the patient became more accepting and less argumentative when given correct information following a confabulation. The authors presented a summary of the seven-step therapy process used in their study.

Treatment for Executive Function and Behavior Deficits

Ylvisaker and Feeney (1998) reported on the use of a well-trained paraprofessional staff to help a TBI patient with a history of alcohol and drug abuse in defining goals, planning, decision-making, and interpreting others' behavior during daily routine activities. Along with waking and eating times, the daily routine involved practice using memory aids, vocational activities for help in getting a job, and group therapy for understanding drug and alcohol abuse. What was once a source of negativism in the patient's daily routine turned into a more positive situation with the help of the staff.

The authors gave examples of negative daily encounters (e.g., waking the patient up and ordering him to participate in the day's activities, which resulted in cursing from the patient and agitation in the staff member) and positive daily encounters (e.g., pleasantly waking the patient who, after dressing and eating breakfast, reviews his goals and with the aid of a staff member, his plans for accomplishing them). Because of this positive interaction with the staff, the once very negative patient increasingly asked for guidance in making a plan and for feedback regarding his perceptions and decisions.

CHAPTER 7

Dysarthria

Motor Speed Disorder

Definition

The condition known as dysarthria can occur alone or can accompany other speech and language disorders. In a seminal study, Darley, Aronson, and Brown (1969a, 1969b, 1975) stated that dysarthria is a collective name for a group of speech disorders that results from disturbances in muscular control over the speech mechanism due to damage of the central or peripheral nervous system.

Dysarthria designates an impairment in oral communication due to paralysis, weakness, or incoordination of the speech musculature. This is in contrast to impairments due to damage in higher centers related to the faulty programming of movement and sequences of movements (apraxia of speech), and to the inefficient processing of linguistic units (aphasia).

Darley et al. (1969a, 1969b, 1975) delineated the various types of dysarthria, each with its own neurologic and speech characteristics. Prior to this perceptual method for delineating the various types of dysarthria, professionals would just use the term dysarthria and provide a description of the speech symptom(s) (see Halpern, Hochberg, & Rees, 1967). The Darley et al. study showed that because speech production follows particular neuroanatomical and neurophysiological

165

pathways, a reference to a specific type of dysarthria can be useful in localizing a lesion. This has clinical value because it serves as a diagnostic tool and can lead to further investigation of the condition.

Darley et al. (1969a, 1969b, 1975) identified 36 different dimensions (symptoms) and 2 overall dimensions (intelligibility and bizarreness) in their dysarthria study. So as not to be overwhelmed by an avalanche of symptoms, the reader is advised to look primarily at those speech symptoms that distinguish one dysarthria from the others. It must be noted that some of the same symptoms may be ranked as most prominent in several dysarthrias and are therefore not considered as reliable differential signs. For example, imprecise consonants were found in all or practically all of the dysarthric subjects in all groups.

In future sections of this chapter, the terms *alternating motion rates* (AMRs) or *diadochokinetic rates* will be used. Both terms refer to checking the speed and consistency of alternating movements of the lips, tongue, and jaw during repetitive articulation.

Symptoms and Etiology

Flaccid Dysarthria

The first type of dysarthria is described as flaccid dysarthria and is, for example, found in the neurologic disorder called bulbar palsy (multiple cranial nerve damage, which can be caused by many of the conditions listed below). All patients in this group displayed evidence of a lower motor neuron lesion, implicating motor units of the cranial nerves involved in speech (V, VII, IX–X, XII). Lesions to lower motor neurons that innervate the respiratory musculature or to the cranial nerves that innervate the speech musculature can result in a flaccid dysarthria.

Weakness of muscle contraction and hypotonia (flaccidity) are the salient features of flaccid dysarthria. It is the only motor speech disorder in which a rapid breakdown of speech can occur after a short period of continuous speaking. Patients with myasthenia gravis can show this deterioration.

Duffy (1995) noted that the etiologies of 107 cases of flaccid dysarthria seen at the Mayo Clinic were as follows: traumatic (34%), composed of surgical trauma (29%) and nonsurgical trauma (5%); neuropathies of undetermined origin (27%); muscle disease (8%); tumor (6%); myasthenia gravis (6%); degenerative (6%); vascular (5%); infectious (3%); anatomic malformation (3%); demyelinating (1%); and other (1%).

Speech Symptoms

Following is a sampling of some of the studies and reports related to the speech symptoms found in flaccid dysarthria. Additional references are noted in the "Diagnosis" and "Therapy" sections of this chapter.

Darley et al. (1969a, 1969b, 1975), in their study of 30 patients with bulbar palsy, found that the most prominent speech deviations (from most to least severe) were hypernasality, imprecise consonants, breathiness (continuous), monopitch, nasal emission, audible inspiration, harsh voice quality, short phrases, and monoloudness.

The speech deviations that best distinguish flaccid dysarthria from the other dysarthrias are described by Darley, et al. (1969a, 1969b, 1975), and by Duffy (1995) in his review of supportive studies in the literature, as *hypernasality*, often coupled with *nasal emission* of air (resulting from incomplete palatopharyngeal closure); *breathiness* that is continuous during phonation (resulting from poor adduction of the vocal folds); *audible inspiration* or stridor on inhalation (resulting from inadequate abduction of the vocal folds); and *short phrases* (resulting from the effect of air wastage through the nose and the need to replenish it frequently).

Respiration Symptoms

Hixon, Putnam, and Sharp (1983) described speech production in a case of flaccid paralysis of the rib cage, diaphragm, and abdomen. The patient was able to combine compensatory neck breathing and glossopharyngeal breathing with other biomechanical and linguistic adaptations into still another functional system for speech production. The authors described the kinematic analysis that took place with this patient.

Hoit, Banzett, Brown, & Loring (1990) used magnetometers to record surface motions of the chest wall in 10 men with traumatic cervical spinal cord injury. The speech characteristics of the subjects showed 3 with reduced loudness, 2 with breathiness, 1 with hypernasality, 1 with rough voice, 1 with imprecise articulation, 2 with short phrases, 1 with long phrases, 1 with long inspiration, and 3 who were normal. Abnormal chest wall activity was attributed mostly to loss of abdominal muscle function. The authors concluded that speech breathing in persons with cervical spinal cord injury may be improved by the use of abdominal binders.

Phonation Symptoms

Aronson (1990) noted that in the flaccid dysarthria of myasthenia gravis, the perceptual laryngeal-phonatory characteristics include the following: a breathy voice quality with weak intensity, a deterioration of phonation during stressful counting or other prolonged speaking activities, and a reduced sharpness of cough after stressful speaking.

The physical appearance of the vocal folds in milder cases may seem normal in structure and function, despite a dysphonia. Absence of findings does exclude presence of milder degrees of bilateral adductor weakness of the vocal folds. In more severe cases, the vocal folds bilaterally may fail to adduct and abduct completely. Bowing of the vocal folds may be present.

Murry (1978) studied 20 subjects with unilateral vocal fold paralysis and found that they had a reduced ability to reach upper pitch ranges. The affected fold becomes flaccid and sluggish, which accounts for the reduced speaking fundamental frequency range. This reduced vocal frequency range may produce a monotone, which is quite often perceived in flaccid dysarthria.

Hammarberg, Fritzell, and Schiratski (1984) analyzed the voice quality of 16 subjects with unilateral paralysis before and after a teflon injection. A perceptual evaluation made after the injection showed that 11 of the 16 subjects made improvement in their voices due to a reduction of breathiness and dysphonia, and in maintaining proper pitch functions. The acoustic measurement of LTAS (long time average spectrum) provided an objective measure of this improvement. Reich and Lerman (1978) found that after a teflon injection in a patient with unilateral vocal fold paralysis there was a general reduction in perceived hoarseness and an enhancement of perceived pleasantness.

Watterson, McFarlane, and Menicucci (1990) studied 9 subjects who had unilateral vocal fold paralysis. Of the 9 subjects, 4 were injected with teflon, 4 were not injected, and 1 was injected but served as a subject in both groups. An additional 3 subjects without vocal fold pathology served as a normal control group. Results showed that subjects in both groups with unilateral vocal fold paralysis (injected and not injected) showed abnormal vibratory characteristics of the vocal folds, whereas the normal subjects showed a more normal picture. Teflon injections with the subjects used in this study proved unsuccessful.

Duffy (1995), in his summary of respiratory and phonatory findings in flaccid dysarthria (based on the literature), confirmed the presence of the respiratory-phonatory symptom of short phrases, and the phonatory symptoms of breathiness and audible inspiration as distinguishing features.

Resonation Symptoms

Garcia and Cannito (1996) reported on a severe flaccid dysarthria patient whose symptoms were primarily characterized by hypernasality, imprecise consonants, short phrases, and breathiness. The study demonstrated that for this dysarthric speaker, speech produced with accompanying communication gestures, with highly predictive sentence content, or with situationally related contexts was more intelligible than speech lacking those characteristics.

Duffy (1995), in his summary of resonatory findings in flaccid dysarthria (based on the literature), confirmed the presence of hypernasality and nasal emission as distinguishing features.

Spastic Dysarthria

The second type of dysarthria is described as spastic dysarthria and is, for example, found in the neurologic disorder called pseudobulbar palsy (bilateral spastic paralysis affecting the bulbar musculature and most commonly caused by multiple or bilateral strokes, and head trauma). The patients in the pseudobulbar group present an upper motor neuron disorder, presumed to involve combined damage to the pyramidal system and to a portion of the extrapyramidal system, both of which arise from the same motor cortex areas. Lesions to upper motor neurons produce spastic muscles that are stiff, move sluggishly through a limited range, and tend to be weak.

Duffy (1995) noted that the etiologies of 107 cases of spastic dysarthria seen at the Mayo Clinic were as follows: vascular (31%); degenerative (30%); traumatic (12%), composed of traumatic brain injury (10%) and surgical trauma (2%); undetermined (12%); demyelinating (6%); tumor (4%); multiple causes (3%); inflammatory (2%); and infectious (1%).

Speech Symptoms

Following is a sampling of some of the studies and reports related to the speech symptoms found in spastic dysarthria. Additional references are noted in the "Diagnosis" and "Therapy" sections of this chapter.

Darley et al. (1969a, 1969b, 1975), in their study of 30 patients with pseudobulbar palsy, found that the most prominent speech deviations (from most to least severe) were imprecise consonants, monopitch, reduced stress, harsh voice quality, monoloudness, low pitch, slow rate, hypernasality, strained-strangled quality, short phrases, distorted vowels, pitch breaks, breathy voice (continuous), and excess and equal stress.

The speech deviations that best distinguish spastic dysarthria from the other dysarthrias are described by Darley, et al. (1969a, 1969b, 1975), and by Duffy (1995) in his review of supportive studies in the literature, as a *strained-strangled voice quality* (resulting from the increased tone of the laryngeal muscles, which causes narrowing of the glottis and increases the resistance to the flow of breath at that level), *slow speech rate,* and *slow and regular alternating motion rates (AMRs)* (the latter two resulting from articulators that move sluggishly with a reduction of range, as well as weakness).

Phonation and Resonation Symptoms

Aronson (1990) noted that in spastic dysarthria, the perceptual laryngeal-phonatory characteristics include the following: a hoarseness or harshness that has a strained-strangled quality, abnormally low pitch accompanied by monopitch, and reduced loudness accompanied by monoloudness. The strained-strangled, harsh voice quality is caused by hyperadduction of the true and false vocal folds, which produces glottic restriction and resistance to the exhalatory air flow.

At rest, the physical appearance of the vocal folds is normal. During speech, the vocal folds can range from looking normal to showing bilateral hyperadduction of the true and false vocal folds.

Duffy (1995), in his summary of phonatory findings in spastic dysarthria (based on the literature), confirmed the presence of *strained-strangled* voice quality as a distinguishing feature.

Articulation and Prosody Symptoms

Hirose, Kiritani, and Sawashima (1982) found a reduced range of articulatory movement in pseudobulbar palsy speech. Ziegler and von Cramon (1986) reported that spastic dysarthric speakers showed a reduction of sound pressure level contrasts in the production of consonants, which may account for imprecise consonants.

Dworkin and Aronson (1986) found that spastic dysarthric speakers had significantly slower rates than normal speakers. Hirose (1986) reported a reduced range of tongue movements and a slowed overall speech rate in spastic dysarthria. Hirose et al. (1982) found a slow rate of speaking in pseudobulbar palsy speech.

Linebaugh and Wolfe (1984) found that spastic dysarthric speakers had significantly longer mean syllable duration than did normal speakers. Portnoy and Aronson (1982) confirmed that spastic dysarthric speakers had a significantly slower and more variable rate in repetition tasks than did normal speakers. Ziegler and von Cramon (1986) reported that spastic dysarthric speakers showed an increase in syllable and word duration, which might account for the slow rate.

Duffy (1995), in his summary of articulatory and prosody findings in spastic dysarthria (based on the literature), confirmed the presence of slow speech rate and slow and regular alternating motion rates (AMRs) as distinguishing features.

Hypokinetic Dysarthria

The third type of dysarthria is described as hypokinetic dysarthria and is, for example, found in the neurologic disorder called Parkinsonism. The extrapyramidal system is responsible for regulating the muscle tone required for posture and for changing position. One of the symptoms of extrapyramidal disease is the reduction of movements, called hypokinesia. The characteristic symptoms of hypokinesia include slowness of movement, limited range of movement, immobility and paucity of movement, rigidity, loss of automatic aspects of movement, and rest tremor.

Parkinsonism is an example of hypokinesia and comes about through damage to the basal ganglia, cortex, and other structures. In particular, the substantia nigra, located in the brain stem, produces a chemical substance called dopamine and sends it to the corpus striatum in the basal ganglia. The corpus striatum turns it into a neural transmitter responsible for its inhibiting influence over muscle tone and movement. Damage to that mechanism is a major cause of Parkinsonism.

In relation to speech, the important feature of hypokinetic disorders is a marked limitation of range of movement. Individualized movements are slow and lack vigor, and often there are hesitations and false starts. Repetitive movements are sometimes slow and at other times very fast and of limited range. It is the only dysarthria in which rapid rate can occur and in which repeated phonemes and palilalia (the involuntary repetition of words and phrases with increasing rate and decreasing loudness) are often found.

Duffy (1995) noted that the etiologies of 107 cases of hypokinetic dysarthria seen at the Mayo Clinic were as follows: degenerative (75%), where Parkinson disease (31%) and Parkinsonism (26%) made up 57% of that total; vascular (10%); undetermined (6%); toxic/metabolic (3%); traumatic (2%); multiple (2%); infectious (1%); and other (1%).

Speech Symptoms

Following is a sampling of some of the studies and reports related to the speech symptoms found in hypokinetic dysarthria. Additional references are noted in the "Diagnosis" and "Therapy" sections of this chapter.

Darley et al. (1969a, 1969b, 1975), in their study of 32 patients with Parkinsonism, found that the most prominent speech deviations (from most to least severe) were monopitch, reduced stress, monoloudness, imprecise consonants, inappropriate silences, short rushes of speech, harsh voice quality, breathy voice (continuous), pitch level, and variable rate.

The speech deviations that best distinguish hypokinetic dysarthria from the other dysarthrias are described by Darley et al. (1969a, 1969b, 1975), and by Duffy (1995) in his review of supportive studies in the literature, as *monopitch, monoloudness, decreased loudness, reduced stress, variable rate, short rushes of speech, overall increases in rate, increased rate within segments, rapid speech AMRs, repeated phonemes,* and *inappropriate silences* (all deviations resulting from a limited range of movement of the musculature, and the rapid rate deviations resulting from the very fast, repetitive movements of a very reduced range that are seen only in Parkinsonism).

Respiration Symptoms

Solomon and Hixon (1993) found that during speech breathing in Parkinson disease, the rib cage and abdominal activities were not as efficient as in normal adults.

Duffy (1995), in his summary of respiratory-phonatory findings in hypokinetic dysarthria (based on the literature), confirmed the presence of decreased loudness as a distinguishing feature.

Phonation Symptoms

Aronson (1990) noted that in hypokinetic dysarthria of Parkinsonism, the perceptual laryngeal-phonatory characteristics include monopitch, reduced stress, monoloudness, reduced loudness, harsh voice quality, and breathy voice quality. Pitch changes require an elevating and lowering of the larynx, a stretching and loosening by contraction and relaxation of the vocal folds, and increase and decrease of infraglottal air pressure. The monopitch voice arises from the rigidity and reduced range of motion of the intrinsic and extrinsic laryngeal muscles needed for these movements.

Necessary for stress and emphasis in normal prosody are the controlled changes of infraglottal air pressure. Because of a reduced range of motion of the abdominal and thoracic muscles used in respiration, the controlled changes in respiration appear diminished in Parkinsonian patients. This loss in emphasis and stress leads to an overall flattening of prosody.

The physical appearance of the vocal folds is normal. Adductor and abductor movements are bilaterally symmetric, but there may be incomplete closure of the vocal folds, which accounts for a breathy voice quality. Reduced loudness and breathiness in the absence of other neurologic signs can indicate early Parkinsonism.

With many Parkinson patients, the administration of the drug L-dopa has caused a lessening of the deviant voice and speech symptoms. Recently, Baker, Ramig, Johnson, and Freed (1997) found that fetal cell transplant (FCT) of dopamine into five individuals with Parkinson disease did not systemically influence their voice and speech production.

Fox and Ramig (1997) observed in 40 patients with idiopathic Parkinson disease that vocal sound pressure level was significantly lower than in normal subjects, and that they rated themselves as significantly more impaired than normal subjects.

Logemann, Fisher, Boshes, and Blonsky (1978) described the frequency of occurrence and the co-occurrence of speech and voice symptoms in 200 Parkinson patients. Of the 200 patients, 178 (89%) had laryngeal dysfunction symptoms, described in descending order of frequency as hoarseness, roughness, breathiness, and tremulousness.

Resonation Symptoms

Hoodin and Gilbert (1989) found that as Parkinsonism deteriorates, the nasal air flow in speakers gets worse. Logemann et al. (1978) found that out of 200 Parkinson patients, 10% were hypernasal.

Articulation and Prosody Symptoms

Logemann et al. (1978) found that out of 200 Parkinson patients, 45% had articulation problems. In a follow-up study, Logemann and Fisher (1981) found a high rate of error on stops and affricates (both due to inadequate tongue elevation to achieve complete closure), and on fricatives (due to inadequate constriction of the airway).

Caligiuri (1989) studied the influence of speaking rate on articulation in Parkinsonian dysarthria and found decreased amplitude, movement time, and speed of labial movements during conversational speech rates, and a reduction of these abnormalities at slower rates. Canter and Van Lancker (1985), in studying a single Parkinson case, found that the rapid rate of this patient's speech was due to a decrease in syllable durations, which resulted from an abnormal shortening of vowels.

Darby, Simmons, and Berger (1984) found that 13 depressed subjects showed reduced stress, monopitch, and monoloudness, which are characteristic symptoms of hypokinetic dysarthria. They compared their results to the Parkinson subjects in the Darley et al. (1975) study. The depressed subjects showed significant improvement after antidepressant medication treatment. The authors suggested that on the basis of the speech signs, a hypokinetic disturbance of the extrapyramidal system exists in depression.

Darkins, Fromkin, and Benson (1988) found that the prosodic loss in Parkinson disease is due to motor control and not to a loss of linguistic knowledge. On the other hand, Natsopoulos et al. (1991), while acknowledging that dysarthria occurs in Parkinson patients, found that a language comprehension disturbance similar to aphasia existed when compared to normal control subjects.

Forrest and Weismer (1995) found that relative to normal geriatic speakers, Parkinsonian speakers produced stressed syllables with reduced movement, amplitude, and velocity. Hammen, Yorkston, and Minifie (1994) observed that synthetic alterations in rate did not increase intelligibility in Parkinsonian dysarthria. Logemann et al. (1978) found that out of 200 Parkinson patients, 20% had rate problems described as syllable repetitions, shortened syllables, lengthened syllables, and excessive pauses.

Duffy (1995), in his summary of articulatory and prosody findings in hypokinetic dysarthria (based on the literature), confirmed the presence of the articulatory symptoms of rapid speech alternating motion rates (AMRs) and repeated phonemes, and the prosody symptoms of monopitch, monoloudness, reduced stress, variable rate, short rushes of speech, overall increase in rate, increased rate within segments, and inappropriate silences as distinguishing features.

Hyperkinetic Dysarthria

The fourth type of dysarthria is described as hyperkinetic dysarthria and is, for example, found in the neurologic disorders called chorea and dystonia. Basically, the hyperkinesias are abnormal involuntary movements, usually due to damage in the basal ganglia control circuit, or occasionally in the cerebellar control circuit or other parts of the extrapyramidal system.

Many involuntary movements are normal (e.g., blinking when the eye is in jeopardy, instantaneous removal of a hand from hot water). Abnormal movements occur in a setting that normally is typified by steady motor movements. The hyperkinesias arise from the failure of the inhibitory functions of the basal ganglia control circuit or the cerebellar control circuit upon the excitatory functions of the motor cortex.

These abnormal involuntary movements are excessive, and their speed can be fast, slow, or both. As a result, some hyperkinesias are called fast (e.g., chorea) and some are called slow (e.g., dystonia). Hyperkinetic dysarthria is a result of the abnormal involuntary muscular movements acting upon the respiratory, phonatory, resonatory, articulatory, and prosody components of speech production. Involuntary movements of the jaw, face, and tongue present during both speech and nonspeech situations are also associated with hyperkinetic dysarthria.

Duffy (1995) noted that the etiologies of 86 cases of hyperkinetic dysarthria seen at the Mayo Clinic were as follows: unknown (59%), where chorea and dystonia were part of that total; toxic/metabolic (17%); degenerative (9%), where Huntington's chorea (5%) and dystonia (1%) were part of that total; multiple (5%), where chorea was part of that total; other (3%); infectious (2%), where Sydenham's chorea made up all of that total; trauma (1%); and vascular (1%).

Huntington's chorea, whose onset occurs in adulthood, is an inherited, progressive, and fatal disease. Sydenham's chorea, whose onset most frequently occurs in childhood, is a noninherited, nonprogressive, and curable disease.

Within the toxic/metabolic etiologic grouping is a condition called tardive dyskinesia. It is quite common for psychiatric patients to undergo long-term ingestion of neuroleptic or antipsychotic medication. These drugs can produce a potentially irreversible disturbance of the central nervous system which is tardive dyskinesia. The characteristics of this condition are abnormal movements within the oral musculature such as sucking and smacking noises, sudden protrusions and retractions of the tongue, rhythmic opening and closing of the mouth, and lateral jaw movements. Portnoy (1979) noted that tardive dyskinesia is manifested in motor speech production as hyperkinetic dysarthria.

Chorea

Speech symptoms. Following is a sampling of some of the studies and reports related to the speech symptoms found in the hyperkinetic dysarthria of chorea. Additional references are noted in the "Diagnosis" and "Therapy" portions of this chapter.

Darley et al. (1969a, 1969b, 1975), in their study of 30 patients with chorea, found that the most prominent speech deviations (from most to least severe) were imprecise consonants, prolonged intervals, variable rate, monopitch, harsh voice quality, inappropriate silences, distorted vowels, excess loudness variation, prolonged phonemes, monoloudness, short phrases, irregular articulatory breakdown, excess and equal stress, hypernasality, reduced stress, and strained-strangled quality.

The speech deviations that best distinguish the hyperkinetic dysarthria of chorea from the other dysarthrias are described by Darley et al. (1969a, 1969b, 1975) and by Duffy (1995), in his review of supportive studies in the literature, as *hypernasality, strained-harshness, transient breathing, articulatory distortions and irregular articulatory breakdowns, loudness variations,* and *sudden forced inspiration or expiration* (all due to the variable and transient pattern of unpredictable movements).

Those speech deviations, along with the speaker's apparent attempt to avoid the interruptions or to compensate for them, result in *prolonged intervals and phonemes, variable rate, inappropriate silences, voice stoppages,* and *excessive or insufficient stress patterns.*

Respiration, phonation, and resonation symptoms. Duffy (1995), in his summary of respiratory findings in the hyperkinetic dysarthria of chorea (based on the literature), confirmed the presence of loudness variations as a distinguishing feature.

Aronson (1990) noted that in the hyperkinetic dysarthria of chorea, the perceptual laryngeal-phonatory characteristics include the following: slow continuous changes in strained-hoarse quality, breathiness, excess loudness variations, voice arrests, monopitch, monoloudness, reduced stress, and excess and equal stress on ordinarily unstressed syllables and words. Sudden uncontrolled movements of the respiratory and laryngeal musculature are responsible for irregular pitch fluctuations and voice arrests, thus producing speech that has a jerky quality. The physical appearance of the vocal folds is normal in structure and function, although there can be intermittent hyperadduction.

Duffy (1995), in his summary of phonatory and resonatory findings in the hyperkinetic dysarthria of chorea (based on the literature), confirmed the presence of the phonatory symptoms of strained-harshness, transient breathiness, sudden forced inspiration or expiration, and voice stoppages, and the resonatory symptom of hypernasality as distinguishing features.

Articulation and prosody symptoms. Duffy (1995), in his summary of articulatory and prosody findings in the hyperkinetic dysarthria of chorea (based on the literature), confirmed the presence of the articulatory symptoms of articulatory distortions and irregular articulatory breakdowns, and the prosody symptoms of prolonged intervals and phonemes, variable rate, inappropriate silences, and excessive or insufficient stress patterns as distinguishing features.

Dystonia

Speech symptoms. Following is a sampling of some of the studies and reports related to the speech symptoms found in the hyperkinetic dysarthria of dystonia. Additional references are noted in the "Diagnosis" and "Therapy" sections of this chapter.

Darley et al. (1969a, 1969b, 1975), in their study of 30 patients with dystonia, found that the most prominent speech deviations (from most to least severe) were imprecise consonants, distorted vowels, harsh voice quality, irregular articulatory breakdown, strained-strangled quality, monopitch, monoloudness, inappropriate silences, short phrases, prolonged intervals, prolonged phonemes, excess loudness variation, reduced stress, voice stoppages, and slow rate. Although below their mean scale value cutoff point of most prominent features, audible inspiration, voice tremor, and alternating loudness occurred with greater frequency than in the other dysarthrias.

The speech deviations that best distinguish the hyperkinetic dysarthria of dystonia from the other dysarthrias are described by Darley et al. (1969a, 1969b, 1975), and by Duffy (1995) in his review of supportive studies in the literature, as *imprecision and irregular breakdowns of articulation, inappropriate variability of loudness and rate, strained harshness, transient breathiness,* and *audible inspiration* (as in chorea, all due to the variable and transient pattern of unpredictable movements).

Those speech deviations, along with the speaker's apparent attempt to avoid the interruptions or to compensate for them, as in chorea, can result in *slow rate, prolonged intervals and phonemes, inappropriate silences,* and *excessive and insufficient stress patterns.*

Respiration and phonation symptoms. Golper, Nutt, Rau, and Coleman (1983) described the speech management program for 10 patients with focal cranial dystonia who showed a slow hyperkinetic dysarthria. Some patients showed some loudness problems, which may be indicative of disturbed breathing movements or a compensation for phonatory stenosis. LaBlance and Rutherford (1991) found that the decreased speech intelligibility in their generalized dystonia subjects was strongly related to decreased breathing patterns.

Aronson (1990) noted that in the hyperkinetic dysarthria of dystonia, the laryngeal-phonatory characteristics include the following: slow, continuous changes in strained-hoarse quality, breathiness, excess loudness variations, voice arrests, monopitch, monoloudness, reduced stress, and excess and equal stress on ordinarily unstressed syllables and words. Sudden uncontrolled adductor and abductor laryngeal spasms can result in strained hoarseness and breathiness, and occasionally paroxysmal inhalatory stridor. The physical appearance of the vocal folds is normal in structure and function, although there can be intermittent hyperadduction.

Duffy (1995), in his summary of respiratory and phonatory findings in the hyperkinetic dysarthria of dystonia (based on the literature), confirmed the presence of the respiratory-phonatory symptom of audible inspiration, the respiratory-phonatory-prosody symptom of inappropriate variability of loudness and rate, and the phonatory symptoms of strained harshness and transient breathiness as distinguishing features.

Articulation and prosody symptoms. Duffy (1995), in his summary of articulatory and prosody findings in the hyperkinetic dysarthria of dystonia (based on the literature), confirmed the presence of the articulatory symptoms of imprecision and irregular breakdowns of articulation, the articulatory-prosody symptom of slow rate, and the prosody symptoms of prolonged intervals and phonemes, inappropriate silences, and excessive and insufficient stress patterns as distinguishing features.

Other Neurologic Disorders

Additional hyperkinetic dysarthrias (Aronson, 1990; Darley et al., 1975; Duffy, 1995) have been found in the following neurologic disorders: organic (essential) voice tremor, palatopharyngolaryngeal myoclonus, Gilles de la Tourette's syndrome, athetosis, spasmodic torticollis, action myoclonus, and spasmodic dysphonia (spastic dysphonia).

Ataxic Dysarthria

The fifth type of dysarthria is described as ataxic dysarthria and is found in neurologic cerebellar disorders. The cerebellum regulates the force, speed, range, timing, and direction of movements arising from the other motor systems. The other motor systems generally start movements in excess of actual need, and the major role of the cerebellum is to dampen or inhibit such overactivity.

Quite often, ataxic dysarthria occurs because of bilateral or generalized damage to the cerebellum. The affected muscles tend to be hypotonic, voluntary movements are slow, and the force, range, timing, and direction of movements are inaccurate. For speech production, the important features of cerebellar disease are inaccuracy of movement, slowness of movement, and hypotonia.

Duffy (1995) noted that the etiologies of 107 cases of ataxic dysarthria seen at the Mayo Clinic were as follows: degenerative (34%), vascular (16%), demyelinating (15%), undetermined (14%), toxic/metabolic (7%), traumatic (6%), inflammatory (5%), tumor (3%), multiple (1%), and other (1%).

Speech Symptoms

Following is a sampling of some of the studies and reports related to the speech symptoms found in ataxic dysarthria. Additional references are noted in the "Diagnosis" and "Therapy" sections of this chapter.

Darley et al. (1969a, 1969b, 1975), in their study of 30 patients with cerebellar lesions, found that the most prominent speech deviations (from most to least severe) were imprecise consonants, excess and equal stress, irregular articulatory breakdown, distorted vowels, harsh voice quality, prolonged phonemes, prolonged intervals, monopitch, monoloudness, excess loudness variations, and voice tremor.

The speech deviations that best distinguish ataxic dysarthria from the other dysarthrias are described by Darley et al. (1969a, 1969b, 1975), and by Duffy (1995) in his review of supportive studies in the literature, as *irregular articulatory breakdowns, irregular speech AMRs* (both resulting from inaccurate direction of movement and dysrhythmia of repetitive movement of the articulators), *excess and equal stress* (resulting from slowness of individual and repetitive movements that places stress on all syllables in a word, including those that are normally produced in an unstressed manner), *distorted vowels* (resulting from inaccurate direction of movement and dysrhythmia of repetitive movement of the articulators), and *prolonged phonemes* (resulting from slowness of individual and repetitive movements of the articulators).

Respiration and Phonation Symptoms

Murdoch, Chenery, Stokes, and Hardcastle (1991) found that respiratory abilities were reduced in speakers with cerebellar disease. These subjects had reduced vital capacities and had a breakdown in the coordination of the rib cage and abdomen while speaking. In particular, these irregularities affected their prosody.

Aronson (1990) noted that in ataxic dysarthria, the perceptual laryngeal-phonatory characteristics include frequently normal phonation; but others can have harsh voice quality, monopitch, monoloudness, excess and equal stress on ordinarily unstressed words or syllables, excess loudness, bursts of loudness, and coarse voice tremor. The physical appearance of the vocal folds is normal in structure and function.

Murry (1984) found that Friedreich's ataxia involves more explosive speech than cerebellar ataxia. Phonatory characteristics are more bizarre, in that there is a rough or harsh quality along with a strained-strangled quality.

Articulation and Prosody Symptoms

Ackerman, Hertrich, and Scharf (1995) found that cerebellar patients had an impaired ability to increase muscular forces in order to produce articulatory gestures of short duration. In a study by Hirose, Kiritani, Ushijima, and Sawashima (1978), electromyography (EMG) findings showed physiological evidence of inconsistency in the articulatory movement of an ataxic dysarthric subject. This pattern seems to be compatible with the characteristic of irregular articulatory breakdown in ataxic dysarthria.

However, Sheard, Adams, and Davis (1991) found that in ratings of ataxic dysarthric speech samples with varying intelligibility, judges agreed mostly on imprecise consonants, excess and equal stress, and harsh voice. They agreed, but less so, on distorted vowels and irregular articulatory breakdown.

Dworkin and Aronson (1986) noted the slowness of speech AMRs in ataxic dysarthric subjects. Gentil (1990) described slow speech rate and slow speech AMRs in 14 subjects with Friedreich's disease. Linebaugh and Wolfe (1984) found that ataxic dysarthric subjects had significantly longer mean syllable duration than did normal subjects. Portnoy and Aronson (1982) observed that ataxic dysarthric subjects had a significantly slower and more variable rate in repetition tasks than normal subjects.

Duffy (1995), in his summary of articulatory and prosody findings in ataxic dysarthria (based on the literature), confirmed the presence of the articulatory symptoms of irregular articulatory breakdowns and irregular speech alternating motion rates (AMRs), the articulatory-prosody symptoms of distorted vowels and prolonged phonemes, and the prosody symptom of excess and equal stress as distinguishing features.

Unilateral Upper Motor Neuron (UUMN) Dysarthria

A sixth type of dysarthria has been studied and reviewed by Duffy (1995) and is called unilateral upper motor neuron (UUMN) dysarthria. The most common cause of this dysarthria is stroke, followed by tumors, and then trauma that can damage upper motor neurons unilaterally.

The outstanding speech characteristics of UUMN dysarthria are imprecise consonants and irregular articulatory breakdown. Harshness, reduced loudness, and mild hypernasality are present in some cases.

Mixed Dysarthria

A seventh type of dysarthria is described as mixed dysarthria and is, for example, found in the neurologic disorder called amyotrophic lateral sclerosis (ALS). In ALS there is a progressive degeneration of both upper and lower motor neurons. Damage to these neurons produces symptoms from both systems, although the appearance of one or the other may predominate depending on the stage of the disease.

Symptoms of upper motor neuron damage (spastic paralysis, hypertonia, hyperreflexia, little or no atrophy, no fasciculations, etc.) are present unless the symptoms of lower motor neuron damage (flaccid paralysis, hypotonia, hyporeflexia, marked atrophy, fasciculations, etc.) predominate. The important features of ALS are weakness of the musculature, very slow production of single and repetitive movements, and reduced range of motion.

Duffy (1995) noted that the etiologies of 300 cases of mixed dysarthria seen at the Mayo Clinic were as follows: degenerative (63%), out of which ALS accounted for 41%; vascular (12%); demyelinating (6%); traumatic (5%); tumor (4%); undetermined (4%); multiple causes (4%); toxic/metabolic (1%); and inflammatory (1%).

Speech Symptoms

Following is a sampling of some of the studies and reports related to the speech symptoms found in ALS. Additional references are noted in the "Diagnosis" and "Therapy" sections of this chapter.

Darley et al. (1969a, 1969b, 1975), in their study of 30 patients with ALS, found that the most prominent speech deviations (from the most to the least severe) were imprecise consonants, hypernasality, harsh voice quality, slow rate, monopitch, short phrases, distorted vowels, low pitch, monoloudness, excessive and equal stress, prolonged intervals, reduced stress, prolonged phonemes, strained-strangled quality, breathiness, audible inspiration, inappropriate silences, and nasal emission.

The speech deviations that best distinguish the mixed dysarthria (flaccid and spastic) in ALS from the other dysarthrias are described by Darley et al. (1969a, 1969b, 1975), and by Duffy (1995) in his review of supportive studies in the literature, as *labored and very slowly produced speech with short phrases and intervals between words and phrases, grossly defective articulation,* (both resulting from articulators that move sluggishly with a reduction of range, as well as weakness) *short phrases* and *intervals between words and phrases,* (resulting from air wastage due to inefficient valving of the vocal folds, the palatopharyngeal area, and the oral area), *marked hypernasality* (resulting from incomplete palatopharyngeal closure), *severe harshness and strained-strangled quality* (resulting from hyperadduction of the vocal folds, which produces glottic restriction and resistance to exhalatory air flow), and *monopitch and monoloudness* (resulting from restricted range of movement of the speech muscles where normal peaks of accent cannot be attained).

Respiration, Phonation, and Resonation Symptoms

Putnam and Hixon (1984), in their study of motor neuron disease patients, found that chest wall muscle weakness produced low lung volume, which resulted in reduced loudness and short phrases. Mulligan et al. (1994) found a greater decrease in forced vital capacity in dysarthric patients with ALS than in nondysarthric patients.

Aronson (1990) noted that in mixed dysarthria of ALS, the perceptual laryngeal-phonatory characteristics include hoarseness or harshness having a strained-strangled quality resulting from hyperadduction of the true and false vocal folds, and a "wet" or "gurgly" sounding hoarseness due to accumulation of saliva on the vocal folds because of a reduced frequency of swallowing. In addition, a rapid tremor or flutter is noted on vowel prolongation. If there is a strong flaccid component, a breathy voice is present due to hyperadduction of the vocal folds. Monopitch and monoloudness can be present, and loudness can be reduced. Audible inhalation can also be present.

The physical appearance of the vocal folds is normal. The vocal folds appear to adduct normally, or may hyperadduct along with the false vocal folds if the prime component is spasticity. Adduction of the vocal folds may be bilaterally symmetric, or one vocal fold may adduct less than the other. The vocal folds may adduct or abduct with less than normal excursions if there is a prime flaccid component.

Kent et al. (1991) attributed hypernasality and harshness as major characteristics in the breakdown of intelligibility in a single ALS patient. Renout, Leeper, Bandur, and Hudson (1995) found reduced and aperiodic vocal fold diadochokinesis in 12 ALS subjects with bulbar, and 14 ALS subjects with nonbulbar signs of the disease.

Duffy (1995), in his summary of phonatory and resonatory findings in the mixed (flaccid and spastic) dysarthria of ALS (based on the literature), confirmed the presence of the phonatory symptoms of severe harshness and strained-strangled quality, the phonatory-resonatory-articulatory symptom of labored and very slowly produced speech with short phrases and intervals between words and phrases, and the resonatory symptom of hypernasality as distinguishing features.

Articulation and Prosody Symptoms

DePaul and Brooks (1993) found that impairment of the tongue was the most critical feature when compared to impairment of the lips and jaw in ALS speakers. Dworkin, Aronson, and Mulder (1980) concluded that dysarthric patients with ALS had lower tongue force than normal subjects. Negative correlations existed between tongue force and severity of articulation. Langmore and Lehman (1994) also found that impairment of the tongue was more crucial than impairment of the jaw and lips in ALS subjects.

Kent et al. (1990) studied the speech intelligibility in men with ALS. They found that the most disrupted phonetic features involved phonatory function (voicing contrast), velopharyngeal valving, place and manner of articulation for lingual consonants, and regulation of tongue height for vowels. Those five features correlated highly with intelligibility. In a follow-up study, Kent et al. (1992) concluded that women with ALS showed results similar to men with ALS, with the exception that men were more likely to have impairments of voicing with syllables in the initial position.

Kent et al. (1991) found that imprecise consonants were a major characteristic in the breakdown of intelligibility in a single ALS patient. Mulligan et al. (1994) found slower diadochokinetic rates and decreased intelligibility in dysarthric patients with ALS than in nondysarthric patients. Samlan and Weismer (1995) looked at articulatory precision and rhythmic consistency as part of a diadochokinetic evaluation, and their relationship to overall speech intelligibility in 15 men with ALS. They found that diadochokinetic judgment was weakly related to overall speech intelligibility in their subjects.

Riddel, McCauley, Mulligan, and Tandan (1995) studied the phonetic breakdown of 29 patients (18 women and 11 men) with early ALS. They found that voicing errors, vowel distortions, longer vowel durations, and contrast errors involving fricatives versus affricates and alveolar fricatives versus palatal fricatives were the significant features of phonetic breakdown in early ALS. They noted that the men appeared more vulnerable to this breakdown than did the women. Turner, Tjaden, and Weismer (1995) found that vowel space area was an important component of global estimates of speech intelligibility in 9 ALS subjects.

Dworkin, Aronson, and Mulder (1980) found that dysarthric patients with ALS had slower syllable repetitions than normal subjects. Negative correlations existed between syllable rate and severity of articulation in ALS. Turner and Weismer (1993) concluded that dysarthric speakers with ALS had more difficulty in changing speaking rate than did normal subjects.

Duffy (1995), in his summary of articulatory and prosody findings in the mixed dysarthria (flaccid and spastic) of ALS (based on the literature), confirmed the presence of the articulatory symptom of grossly defective articulation and the prosody symptoms of monopitch and monoloudness.

Other Neurologic Disorders

Additional mixed dysarthrias have been found in the following neurologic disorders:

Multiple sclerosis (MS) (Darley, et al. 1975; Darley, Brown, and Goldstein, 1972) most frequently showed a mixture of ataxic and spastic dysarthric components, although each component can be present alone. Because of the unpredictability of MS, in some patients any other single type of dysarthria or other mixture can be present. Hartelius, Buder, and Strand (1997) reported on the long-term phonatory instability of 20 individuals with MS, including those who had ataxic and spastic components.

Wilson's disease (Berry, Darley, Aronson, and Goldstein, 1974; Darley et al., 1975; Day and Parnell, 1987) showed ataxic, spastic, and hypokinetic dysarthric components in different mixtures, although each component can be present alone in some patients.

Shy-Drager syndrome (Linebaugh, 1979) showed ataxic, hypokinetic, and spastic dysarthric components in different mixtures, although each component can be present alone in some patients.

Progressive supranuclear palsy (reviewed by Duffy, 1995) most frequently showed hypokinetic and spastic dysarthric components alone or as a mixture. However, ataxic dysarthric components, typically in combination with hypokinetic or spastic components, can also be present in some patients.

Friedreich's ataxia (reviewed by Duffy, 1995) showed ataxic dysarthria as the most frequently occurring type, followed by spastic dysarthria, and then by scattered other types. The most common mixture would be that of ataxic and spastic components.

Olivopontocerebellar atrophy (reviewed by Duffy, 1995) showed ataxic, spastic, or flaccid dysarthric components, or various mixtures of all three. This atrophy also may be associated with Parkinsonian features, so there is a possibility that a hypokinetic dysarthric component may be present.

Undetermined Dysarthria

An eighth type of dysarthria, called undetermined dysarthria (Duffy, 1995), indicates that a neurogenic motor speech disorder is present but that its perceptual symptoms are either very subtle, complicated, or unusual. In that case, a diagnosis of "motor speech disorder, type undetermined" might be warranted.

Diagnosis

Diagnostic procedures for determining dysarthria can involve (a) establishing background information, (b) giving a neurologic evaluation, (c) perceptual evaluation of the speech and voice characteristics, (d) assessing the oral mechanism at rest and during nonspeech activities, and (e) evaluation through instrumentation.

Establishing Background Information and the Neurologic Evaluation

These procedures can be found at the beginning of the "Diagnosis" section of Chapter 3.

Perceptual Evaluation of the Speech and Voice Characteristics

Lass, Ruscello, and Lakawicz (1988) and Lass, Ruscello, Harkins, and Blankenship (1993) found that listener perception of dysarthric speech adversely affected their notion of the speaker's personality and physical appearance. Recently, Garcia and Dagenais (1998) studied the sentence intelligibility of 4 speakers with dysarthria. They found that an audio plus video presentation, rather than an audio-only presentation, enhanced listener understanding for all speakers. They also found that the contributions of relevant signal-independent information (gestures and message predictiveness) were greater for the speakers with more severely impaired intelligibility.

Following are several informal tests used in a perceptual evaluation of dysarthria.

A systematic perceptual evaluation of dysarthria requires a sample of several types of speech and voice production. The clinician should look for the symptoms described under each type of dysarthria. As suggested by Darley et al. (1975), a checklist of dysarthric symptoms might be used as a guideline and form sheet (see Table 7.1). Symptoms can be evaluated according to their intelligibility (clarity) and bizarreness (understandable but varying very much from standard production). A 7-point scale can be used for evaluating each symptom in the checklist (Table 7.1): 1 = normal, 2 = mild, 3 = mild to moderate, 4 = moderate, 5 = moderate to severe, 6 = severe, 7 = very severe to unintelligible.

Table 7.1. Checklist of Dysarthric Symptoms

A. Respiration
   1. reduced loudness ☐
   2. excessive loudness ☐
   3. monoloudness ☐
   4. intermittent loudness ☐
   5. loudness decay ☐
   6. forced inhalation or exhalation ☐
   7. grunt at end of exhalation ☐
   8. loudness level overall ☐

B. Phonation
   1. breathiness ☐
   2. strained-strangled ☐
   3. harshness ☐
   4. hoarseness ☐
   5. pitch breaks ☐
   6. tremors ☐
   7. monopitch ☐
   8. audible inhalation ☐
   9. voice stoppages ☐
  10. pitch level overall ☐

C. Resonance
   1. hypernasality ☐
   2. nasal emission ☐
   3. nasality overall ☐

D. Articulation
   1. distortion, omissions, substitutions, and additions of consonants ☐
   2. distortions, omissions, substitutions, and additions of vowels and diphthongs ☐
   3. articulation level overall ☐

E. Prosody
   1. monotone ☐
   2. excessive and equal stress ☐
   3. inappropriate silences ☐
   4. stress or vocal variety level overall ☐
   5. slow rate ☐
   6. short rushes of speech ☐
   7. rate level overall ☐

AMR alternating motion rate
diadochokenetic rates
Dysarthria * 189
SMR sequential motion rate

The patient can be asked to do the following:

1. Prolong /ah/, /ee/, and /oo/ separately, as long, as clearly, and as steadily as possible. Normal speakers can sustain the vowel /ah/ anywhere from 10 to 34.6 seconds (reviewed by Duffy, 1995).

   Numbers 2, 3, and 4 represent evaluation through alternating motion rate (AMR), which can check the speed and consistency of alternating movements of the lips, tongue, and jaw.

2. Repeat /puh/ as rapidly as possible.

3. Repeat /tuh/ as rapidly as possible.

4. Repeat /kuh/ as rapidly as possible. The AMR for normal speakers for /puh/, /tuh/, and /kuh/ ranges from 5 to 7 repetitions per second, with repetition of /kuh/ somewhat slower (reviewed by Duffy, 1995). Dworkin and Aronson (1986) found that dysarthric speakers showed weaker tongue strength and slower AMR than did normal speakers.

   Number 5 represents evaluation through sequential motion rate (SMR), which can check the rapid movement of one sound to another in sequence.

5. Repeat /puh-tuh-kuh/ as rapidly as possible. The SMR for nominal speakers for /puh-tuh-kuh/ ranges from 3.6 to 7.5 repetitions per second (as reviewed by Duffy, 1995).

6. Repeat "snowman."

7. Repeat "gingerbread."

8. Repeat "impossibility."

Patients can be asked to respond out loud to action pictures, read out loud a phonetically balanced passage (e.g., grandfather passage), and respond out loud to standardized articulation tests or tests used specifically for dysarthria patients.

Tikofsky and Tikofsky (1964) and Yorkston and Beukelman (1980b) proposed that dysarthric patients read lists of words; based upon their intelligibility, the clinician can determine degrees of impairment. In a later study, Yorkston and Beukelman (1981b) found that speaking rate and speech intelligibility can distinguish mildly dysarthric from normal speakers.

Beukelman and Yorkston (1980a) also found that speech pathologists overestimated intelligibility of dysarthric speech, possibly because
of familiarity with the passage. In a later study, Yorkston and Beukelman (1983) found that familiarization with the dysarthric speaker did
not increase intelligibility scores.

Kent, Weismer, Kent, and Rosenbek (1989) created a word intelligibility test for use with dysarthric speakers. Their test is designed to
examine 19 acoustic-phonetic contrasts that are likely to (a) identify
dysarthric impairment, and (b) contribute significantly to speech intelligibility.

The following are two formalized tests used in a perceptual evaluation of dysarthria.

Assessment of Intelligibility of Dysarthric Speech (Yorkston and Beukelman, 1981a) is a tool for quantifying single-word intelligibility, sentence
intelligibility, and speaking rate of adult and adolescent dysarthric
speakers. Measures of speech intelligibility and speaking rate serve as
an index of dysarthric severity, thus enabling the clinician to rank different dysarthric speakers, compare performance of a single dysarthric
speaker to normal performance, and monitor changing performance
over time.

The Frenchay Dysarthria Assessment (Enderby, 1983) is another test
that can be used for evaluation of dysarthria. This test is divided into 11
sections: Reflex, Respiration, Lips, Jaw, Palate, Larynx, Tongue, Intelligibility, Rate, Sensation, and Influencing Factors (hearing, sight, teeth,
language, mood). The patient is asked to perform designated tasks (e.g.,
"Say 'ah' for as long as possible" and "Count to 20 as quickly as possible") on 8 of the sections. Scoring is based on a patient's second
attempt at each task; a 9-point rating scale is used. This examination
was designed for use in categorically diagnosing dysarthria. Sample
profiles are provided for five types of dysarthria: upper motor neuron
lesion, mixed upper and lower motor neuron lesions, extrapyramidal
disorders, cerebellar dysfunction, and lower motor neuron lesion.

Assessing the Oral Mechanism at Rest and During Nonspeech Activities

Duffy (1995) noted that examination of the oral mechanism at rest and
during nonspeech activities can provide confirmatory evidence and
information about the size, strength, symmetry, range, tone, sturdiness,

speed, and accuracy of orofacial structures and movements. He described in detail how observation of the face (lips, mouth, cheeks, eyes), jaw, tongue, velopharynx, larynx, and respiration are made at rest, during sustained postures and movements, and in response to tests for normal and primitive reflexes.

Assessment procedures of voluntary versus automatic nonspeech movements of the speech mechanism are described when nonverbal oral apraxia is a possibility.

The following are two formalized tests for assessment of the oral mechanism at rest and during nonspeech activities.

The Dworkin-Culatta Oral Mechanism Examination (Dworkin & Culatta, 1980) includes 10 subtests that evaluate facial appearance, circumoral musculature, dentition and gingiva, hard palate, velopharyngeal mechanism, tongue, laryngeal mechanism, and oral and speech praxes. After administering the full examination, abnormal signs are noted on a checklist. The signs are then compared to the error profiles of 23 conditions. Each of the 23 conditions is described on the basis of site of neurologic involvement (e.g., extrapyramidal system, basal ganglia) or of anatomical abnormality (e.g., velum, tongue), and the tests and subcategories of tests that yielded the abnormal signs. The protocols also contain six sample reports of patients who manifested dysarthrias of the spastic, flaccid, hyperkinetic, and mixed spastic-ataxic types; oral apraxia and apraxia of speech; and physiologic disorders associated with structural and physiological abnormalities.

The Oral Speech Mechanism Screening Examination, Revised Edition (St. Louis & Ruscello, 1987) provides a quick method for performing oral speech mechanism examinations. Requiring 5 to 10 minutes to administer, this test examines the lips, tongue, jaw, teeth, hard palate, soft palate, pharynx, velopharyngeal functions, breathing, and diadochokinetic rates.

Three interpretations are possible for each of the structures or functions evaluated: normal, abnormal with referral to another specialty for additional assessment, and further testing to verify and more fully describe the disorder. Separate numerical subscores for structure and function, as well as a total score, permit comparison of individual clients with normal speakers. Included in the protocols is a detailed description of the importance of each structure to speech production, its appearance, and typical deviations.

Evaluation Through Instrumentation

Simmons (1983) performed cineradiographic and spectrographic analysis to study the speech production of a subject who presented the classic neurological signs of cerebellar lesion and had speech characteristics similar to those that have been reported for ataxic dysarthria. Barlow, Cole, and Abbs (1983) described a head-mounted, lip-jaw movement transduction system for the study of motor speech disorders, and Barlow and Abbs (1983) further described the use of force transducers for the evaluation of labial, lingual, and mandibular motor impairments.

Hixon et al. (1983) discussed the use of a kinematic procedure in measuring speech production in a patient with flaccid paralysis of the rib cage, diaphragm, and abdomen. O'Dwyer, Neilson, Guitar, Quinn, and Andrews (1983) noted the use of EMG in evaluating the activity of orofacial and mandibular muscles of dysarthric subjects during non-speech tasks.

Barlow and Burton (1990) and Wood, Hughes, Hayes, and Wolfe (1992) studied the use of lip force as a neuromotor assessment tool. Wit, Maassen, Gabreels, and Thoonen (1993) proposed the use of Maximum Performance Tests, which include maximum sound prolongation, fundamental frequency range, and maximum repetition rate as tools for detecting spastic dysarthria.

Netsell (1994) noted that the best candidates for instrumentation testing and special procedures are patients with severe dysarthria who have unintelligible speech and may have the potential to regain intelligibility. Netsell stated that the best instruments are (a) those involving aerodynamics, where changes in air flow and pressure can be measured by *rhinometers*, and lung volume levels and air expired during speech by motorized *spirometers*; (b) *video-fluoroscopy*, which is used in swallowing detection, to visualize the lips, tongue, jaw, and velopharynx during speech (if a microphone is added, speech can be seen and heard at the same time); and (c) *videonasoendoscopic* systems, which can be used to see the superior aspects of the velopharynx and the larynx.

Therapy

The first goal of therapy is to inform the patient and the caretaker(s) about the nature and the consequences of the disorder.

The dysarthric patient has a motor speech disorder that involves paralysis within the vocal tract. The speech components affected can involve respiration, phonation, resonation, articulation, and prosody in any combination. Typically, thinking abilities are normal or near normal, and language should be normal.

Prognosis

Netsell (1984) suggested six factors that influence treatment outcome with dysarthric patients:

1. *Neurologic status and history.* Bilateral subcortical or brain stem lesions, and degenerative diseases such as ALS offer the poorest prognosis. Love, Hagerman, and Taimi (1980) found that cerebral palsy subjects with more frequent dysphagic symptoms tended to present lower scores of overall speech proficiency and poor articulation scores. Neurologic history should be observed to see if developmental (e.g., cerebral palsy) or acquired dysarthria is present. Treatment procedures geared specifically to the cause would offer a better prognosis.

2. *Age.* Persons experiencing neurological insults during the development of the neocortical system might be expected to have, or to develop, better speech motor skills than those in whom the lesion occurred at a later age. The implication is that intact reticulolimbic systems can support the more innate early motor skills. Younger children have a better chance to "grow out of" their lesions than adults. Elderly patients are negatively affected by age.

3. *"Automatic" adjustments.* In response to a lesion, automatic adjustments can be adaptive or maladaptive, intended or unintended, and reactive or "obligatory" (always the same). Incorporating automatic adjustments that are useful and minimizing those that are not offers a better prognosis.

4. *Treatment effects.* Treatment, especially combined (speech, medical, physical, behavioral) is better than no therapy or noncoordinated therapy.

5. *Personality and intelligence.* Those who were optimistic and purposeful before injury have a better prognosis than those who were not. Understanding premorbid levels of intelligence should aid in therapy.

6. *Support systems.* Treatment is enhanced if support is given by "significant others" and if the prospects for making contributions to society, however modest, are realistic.

The second goal of therapy is to provide the appropriate treatment approaches and techniques.

Efficacy of Therapy for Dysarthria

Yorkston (1996) reviewed a number of treatment efficacy studies of dysarthria. She found that several treatment techniques have been successfully applied to dysarthria caused by Parkinson disease, stroke and traumatic brain injury, cerebral palsy, and some other etiologies.

In Parkinson disease, the treatment studies ranged from retrospection to group to individual, with programs designed to improve voice loudness, intonation, articulation, and phonation. In the late 1960s and early 1970s, the broad-based speech improvement programs seemed to bring improvement during the treatment session, but these gains were not maintained outside the clinical setting. In the late 1970s and early 1980s, success was reported in the use of pacing boards and portable delayed auditory feedback devices.

During the 1980s, studies designed to improve respiration, voice, articulation, rate, intonation, intelligibility, and prosody showed success during the treatment session and some maintenance of progress. In the 1990s, several well controlled group studies showed that treatment focusing on respiratory-phonatory function is more effective in changing the speech of patients with Parkinson disease than is treatment focusing on respiratory function alone.

For stroke and traumatic brain injury, Yorkston (1996) noted that group studies of persons with dysarthria following brain injury are not common because the pattern and severity of the dysarthria vary so extensively in this population. A number of case studies have shown that effective treatment for dysarthric patients includes physiologic approaches (neuromuscular exercises), feedback of acoustic information, and rate control and breath patterning. Studies have shown that important changes in speech can occur many years post-onset of TBI and suggest that long-term follow-up is necessary for brain-injured individuals with severe dysarthria.

Devices such as alphabet boards and palatal lifts also have been efficacious with dysarthric individuals. Outcomes of these studies are measured in several ways, including improvement in muscle strength or control, reduction in a selected deviant feature (e.g., consonant imprecision), and changes in overall features such as speech intelligibility, speaking rate, or naturalness.

Yorkston (1996) noted that reports on the efficacy of speech treatment for individuals with cerebral palsy are scarce. Some evidence suggests that speakers with cerebral palsy are able to modify their speech behaviors when faced with communication failure, or when using breath-group treatment strategy. Many published reports related to the effectiveness of treatment in cerebral palsy involve application of augmentative and alternative communication. It is beyond the scope of this book to report on the success of treatment using augmentative or alternative communication approaches in individuals with cerebral palsy and dysarthria. For this information, the reader is referred to the review of treatment efficacy in dysarthria by Yorkston (1996).

Concerning other etiologies, Yorkston (1996) noted that effective speech treatments for individuals with amyotrophic lateral sclerosis involved having the patient stay in the community, enhancing the quality of life, and providing modeling and instructions. Treatment effectiveness was also reported for the following types of individuals: in intensive or acute medical care units; with Wilson's disease; with multiple sclerosis; with Moebius syndrome, characterized by bilateral facial paralysis; with progressive nuclear palsy; with Shy-Drager Syndrome; and with oral movement disorders.

General Principles

Darley et al. (1975) suggested the following general principles that underlie therapy for the motor speech disorders:

1. *Compensation.* The patient learns to make maximum use of the remaining potential and to "work around" the impairment that has altered his lifelong speech habits.

2. *Purposeful activity.* The patient learns to do on purpose what she had been doing automatically before. The patient must develop an awareness of where her articulators are and of what they are

doing, of how word sequences fall into phrase groupings, of how breath supply can be coordinated with the onset of speech effort and adjusted to the appropriate phrase units, and of how her voice varies in loudness.

3. *Monitoring.* The patient learns to listen to himself talk (perhaps by listening to tape recordings of his speech performances from time to time), noting specific ways in which he falls short of his standard, whether in audibility, intelligibility, or emphasis.

4. *An early start.* The patient gets a head start in compensation, purposeful activity, and monitoring before her skills have deteriorated and it becomes next to impossible to sustain the effort to speak well.

5. *Motivation.* The patient is reassured that his effort is worthwhile. The clinician plans a sensible sequence of activities graduated in difficulty, with an optimistic manner that encourages the patient to do his best.

Indirect and Direct Treatment

Brookshire (1997) noted that treatment for dysarthria can be indirect, direct, or most likely a combination of the two. Indirect approaches would include sensory stimulation, muscle strengthening, modifying muscle tone, changing the posture and speaking position, and modifying respiration.

The purpose of sensory stimulation is to heighten motor control by increasing the patient's awareness of sensory feedback from the oral mechanism. Stimulation techniques may include brushing, stroking, vibration, or applying ice to the patient's lips, tongue, pharynx, or soft palate. The value of sensory stimulation is still debatable.

The purpose of muscle strengthening is to improve the patient's speech by increasing movements of weakened muscles. Muscle strengthening exercises work best for patients with severe dysarthria, where there is little intelligible speech. For the mild or moderately impaired patient, the value of muscle strengthening is debatable.

Defects in muscle tone can be manifested as hypertonicity (e.g., spastic dysarthria) or as hypotonicity (e.g., flaccid dysarthria). The modification of muscle tone in hypertonicity primarily includes techniques that relax the muscles (e.g., progressive relaxation, chewing exercises). The modification of muscle tone in hypotonicity can include techniques that increase the level of muscle tension (e.g., pushing and pulling exercises).

Changing the posture and speaking position of the patient can sometimes improve his or her speech production. These changes are most beneficial for the weak or flaccid patient who has difficulty sitting up and keeping his or her head in an upright position. Cervical collars, body braces, slings, restraints, girdles, stomach bands, and stomach boards are among the items used to assist the patient in achieving this change.

Modifying respiration capacity is most beneficial for patients with a generalized weakness. Treatment can include postural and positioning adjustments, muscle strengthening of the respiratory muscles, increasing muscle tone with pushing exercises, and controlled exhalation techniques. Rosenbek and LaPointe (1985) presented in full detail the modification procedures for posture, muscle tone, and strength for general purposes, and for respiration, phonation, resonation, and articulation specifically.

Direct treatment procedures involve controlling respiration, phonation, resonation, articulation, and prosody in any combination during speech production. In the following pages are some of the indirect and direct treatment procedures for problems in articulation, hypernasality, strained-strangled voice, breathiness, prosody impairment (varying pitch, controlling rate), and loudness impairment, and for severe dysarthria. In some cases, indirect and direct treatment techniques are combined, and in other cases the entire approach is either direct or indirect. The concept of indirect and direct treatment procedures will be mentioned specifically only in the section dealing with therapy for articulation disorders. However, the concept should apply to all the other forms of therapy for dysarthria.

Articulation

For problems in articulation, mobility and stretching techniques may be used as indirect treatment. Duffy (1995) stated that stretching exercises of the lips, tongue, and jaw may have some effect on increasing range of motion and decreasing spasticity in speech. Because stretching of the articulators is necessarily voluntary and not passive, it may also contribute to increasing strength. Stretching may work best for those with spasticity and rigidity, and the possible strengthening effect of stretching might help some patients with weakness.

It must be noted that vigorous exercises of the articulators are contraindicated for conditions such as myasthenia gravis, where such exercises would produce a further weakening of the musculature (Darley et al., 1975; Rosenbek & LaPointe, 1985).

Duffy (1995) stated that nonspeech strengthening exercises should be used only after ascertaining that weakness is clearly related to the speech impairment. Although there is some controversy concerning the efficacy of strengthening exercises to improve articulation in dysarthric patients (see Duffy, 1995), strengthening exercises have been recommended by Dworkin (1991) and Solomon and Stierwalt (1995).

The following exercises numbered 1–5, 7–11, and 13–17 are examples of mobility and stretching activities. Exercises numbered 6 (lips) and 12 (tongue) are examples of strengthening activities. Exercises numbered 1–17 are examples (Kilpatrick & Jones, 1977) of indirect treatment. Exercises 18–21 are examples of direct treatment using alternating motion rate activities.

A mirror should be used to do these exercises. The patient should do each exercise 5 times (less if necessary) and gradually, over a number of lessons, work up to 10 times. All exercises should be done 3 times (less if necessary) a day. The clinician should demonstrate each exercise.

1. Open and close mouth slowly; be sure lips are fully closed; hold, relax, and repeat.

2. Pucker lips, as for a kiss; hold, relax, and repeat.

3. Spread lips into a big smile; hold, relax, and repeat.

4. Pucker, hold, smile, hold; relax and repeat.

5. Open mouth, then try to pucker with mouth wide open, don't close jaw; hold, relax, and repeat.

6. Close lips tightly and press together; hold, relax, and repeat.

7. Close lips; suck tongue as if it were candy.

8. Open mouth and stick out tongue; be sure tongue comes straight out of your mouth and doesn't go off to the side; hold, relax, and repeat. Work toward sticking tongue out farther each day, but still pointing straight ahead.

9. Stick out tongue and move it slowly from corner to corner of your lips; hold it in each corner; relax and repeat. Be sure tongue actually touches each corner each time.

10. Stick out tongue and try to reach chin with the tongue tip; hold at farthest point; relax, repeat.

11. Stick out tongue and try to reach nose with the tongue tip; pretend to lick a popsicle or clean off some jelly from top lip (don't use bottom lip or fingers as helpers); give it a good stretch; hold, relax, and repeat.

12. Using tongue blade or spoon, stick out tongue; hold spoon against the tip of tongue and try to push the spoon even farther away with tongue while hand is holding the spoon steadily in place (hold the spoon like a popsicle or a sucker upright and not in mouth); relax and repeat.

13. Stick out tongue; pretend to lick a sucker, moving the tongue tip from near the chin to near the nose; go slowly and use as much movement as possible; relax and repeat.

14. Stick tongue out and pull it back, then repeat as quickly as you can; repeat.

15. Move tongue from corner to corner as quickly as you can; repeat.

16. Move tongue all around lips in a circle as quickly and as completely as you can, touching all of both upper lip and corner, lower lip and corner, in circle; repeat.

17. Open and close mouth as quickly as possible; be sure lips close each time; repeat.

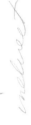

18. Say "mah-mah-mah-mah" as quickly and accurately as you can without losing the "mah" sound; be sure there's an /m/ and an /ah/ each time.

19. Say "lah-lah-lah-lah" as quickly and accurately as possible; be sure there's an /l/ and an /ah/ each time; repeat.

20. Say "kah-kah-kah-kah" as quickly and accurately as you can; be sure there's a /k/ and an /ah/ each time; repeat.

21. Say "kahlah-kahlah-kahlah" as quickly and accurately as you can; be sure there's a /k/ and an /ah/ and an /l/ and an /ah/ each time; repeat.

To round out the above list, one can add exaggerated chewing exercises (indirect treatment) and production of sequential motion rate exercises (direct treatment) of /puh-puh-puh/tuh-tuh-tuh/kuh-kuh-kuh/, and /puh-tuh-kuh/. Occasionally, the above exercises will have to be adapted in some way. For example, one dysarthria patient did not want to smile when asked because she was in no mood to smile. She was gloomy and depressed about her condition and related matters, and could not bring herself to produce even the faintest of smiles. However, when asked to "Show me your teeth," she did, and one would think the sun had burst through the clouds.

Therapy that focuses on phoneme production (direct treatment) can include the following:

1. The phonetic placement method of describing the correct manner and place of articulation, and the correct voiced and voiceless components of target phoneme production uses both visual and verbal instruction.

2. The motokinesthetic approach, which is the manual manipulation of the articulators to produce the correct sound, can also be employed. This approach should be used with some caution because a study by Creech, Wertz, and Rosenbek (1973) showed dysarthric patients to be somewhat deficient in stereognostic abilities.

3. The phonetic derivation method (Rosenbek, 1985) achieves the correct production of sounds from intact nonspeech or speech gestures. For example, biting the lower lip produces /f, v/, puckering the lips produces /oo, oh, aw, w/, smiling produces /ee, eh/, yawning produces /ah, uh/, and wiping one's mouth produces /m, p, b/.

4. Using the above three approaches, the sound is worked on in isolation (most likely with the severe dysarthric patient) and then with real words or with nonsense syllables (e.g., "ah, ay, ee, aw, oh, oo"), unconnected syllables (e.g., "s-ah"), and in

connected form (e.g., "sah"). After this is achieved, the sound is employed in the initial, final, medial, and blend positions in words, phrases, sentences, and eventually controlled conversations.

5. Once the patient has achieved some success in producing consonant sounds, the use of minimal contrasts in single words (e.g., "tea–key"), phrases (e.g., "tan coat"), and sentences (e.g., "Ted can tell Kay about the two cars") can be used to bolster each individual consonant and to differentiate between consonants that are close. Keith and Thomas (1989) provided practice material for the vowels, diphthongs, and consonants for contrast purposes. Listed below are examples of contrasting pairs of words and phrases.

tea–key	tea cup
till–kill	Tim came
ten–Ken	tell Kay
tan–can	tan coat
tall–call	tall cow
top–cop	Tom cat
take–cake	take care
two–coo	two keys
tub–cub	tough call
toad–code	toll call

6. Another technique to achieve overall intelligibility requires the patient to read aloud lists of single words, sentences, or paragraphs; describe a picture; or engage in controlled conversation. The clinician can either face the patient or not, and try to discern the intelligibility of what the patient is saying. If the patient is unclear, imitation of the clinician can be effective in producing intelligibility. This technique can also be used with patients who have loudness, phonatory, nasality, rhythm, or rate problems.

7. Slowing the rate of speech is another procedure that might increase intelligibility in articulation (see Berry, 1984; Darley et al., 1975). Yorkston, Hummen, Beukelman, and Traynor

(1990) found that slow rate helped sentence but not phoneme intelligibility in dysarthric speakers. They also found that slowed rate affected the naturalness in normal speakers, but not so much in dysarthric speakers. In addition to slowing the rate of speech, Darley et al. (1975) advocated consonant exaggeration (e.g., "important, because") and a syllable-by-syllable approach (e.g., "af-ter sup-per, when-ev-er pos-si-ble") as a means of increasing intelligibility in articulation.

Medical, Pharmacological, and Prosthetic Management

Duffy (1995) reviewed the use of the following as aids in articulation therapy: surgical management (neural anastomosis, which with dysarthric patients usually involves connecting the XII nerve to the damaged VII nerve to restore function; botox injections for treatment of hemifacial spasm, spasmodic torticollis, and oral mandibular dystonia), pharmacological management, and prosthetic management (bite block made of acrylic or putty material that is custom fitted to be held between the lateral upper and lower teeth to inhibit uncontrolled jaw movements).

Hypernasality

The following are some suggestions for therapy.

1. Because hypernasality is caused by insufficient movement of the velum, one intervention approach involves stimulating the muscles of the soft palate:
   A. Sip through a straw with the other end sealed.
   B. Produce a very long (pull-in) kiss with a loud smack at the end.
   C. Perform pushing exercises (Froeschels, Kastein, & Weiss, 1955), which require the patient to push with both arms and hands down against a table top, upward under a table, hand against hand, or in a parallel downward motion against the air. This motion is accompanied by the /ah/ sound. With the sudden voluntary contraction of one group of muscles, other muscle groups tend to con-

tract, reinforcing the function of the first group (muscles of the soft palate).

D. Repeat /ah/ strongly and rapidly without pushing.

E. Exercise for the back of the tongue (e.g., "kah, kay, kee" and "ahk, ayk, eek") can also be employed in stimulating the muscles of the soft palate; here, the production of lin- guavelar consonants provides the stimulation to the soft palate.

2. Another technique for reducing hypernasality involves directing the air stream through the oral cavity:

A. Straws (putting a straw in water and blowing bubbles), bubble pipes, oral-nasal cardboard platforms, ping-pong balls, horns, whistles, musical instruments, pinwheels, candles, balloons, feathers, and paper have all been used to refocus the direction of the air stream.

B. A sheet of paper with a hole or bull's-eye in the center can be held close to the patient's lips. The patient is instructed to hit the hole or bull's-eye with the /oo/ sound pro- duced through the oral cavity. The clinician slowly moves the paper away as the patient keeps phonating. The paper can be moved only if the patient produces the cor- rect /oo/ sound through the oral cavity. This technique might be applicable as a breathing exercise in that it helps to prolong the breath stream.

Both the techniques of stimulating the muscles and of directing the air stream should be instituted with some caution, because some studies reviewed by Duffy (1995) have shown that these procedures may have little or no value in reducing hypernasality.

3. Tongue exercises (rotation, in and out) and lip exercises (pursing, puckering, retracting, biting down or up) are used to achieve flexibility. Also, because a raised mandible and retracted tongue tend to isolate the oral cavity, thereby increasing the hypernasality, tongue and lip exercises are used to prevent such movement. Appropriate exercises should open up the oral cavity as a resonator and combat the patient's attempts to retract the tongue or raise the mandible in an effort to reduce hypernasality.

Strained-Strangled Voice

The problem of strained-strangled voice is due to overadduction of the vocal folds. Therefore, a major thrust of therapy is attaining soft and easy onset of phonation. Suggestions for therapy include the following:

1. The yawn-sigh technique, in which the patient is taught to produce phonation in an easy, relaxed yawn. The rationale for this technique is that yawning opens up the entire vocal tract, thereby cutting down on hyperadduction of the vocal folds. Initially, the patient yawns and releases a sigh on exhalation.

2. Another technique is to teach the patient to initiate phonation with the phoneme /h/, since this phoneme is produced with the vocal folds abducted, and can eventually be employed to initiate the production of words and phrases.

3. Relaxation exercises centered around the head and neck area can also be used. In this instance, the patient imagines that his head is a heavy iron ball and lets it drop on his chest. Then he slowly rotates his head in a front-to-back motion and emits phonation while rotating his head. The relaxation of the head and neck area should help bring about easy onset of phonation.

   Rubow, Rosenbek, Collins, and Celesia (1984) reported that EMG biofeedback as a method for producing relaxation, successfully reduced the strained-strangled quality in a patient with hemifacial spasm and dysarthria. Nemec and Cohen (1984) found that EMG biofeedback was an effective treatment technique in a case of hypertonic spastic dysarthria.

4. Chewing exercises, which are based on the concept of eating, can be used for attaining relaxation and proper muscular tonus in the vocal tract. In a graduated series of steps, the patient is taught exaggerated chewing movements without and then with phonation. Using these movements, the patient progresses from single word phonation to conversational speech. Eventually, the exaggerated movements are reduced to where she can chew mentally. Chewing exercises

are described in detail by their originator, Froeschels (1952), and by Boone (1983).

Chiefly for spastic dysarthria, Aten (1984) suggested that all movements should be relaxed and slow, to avoid triggering the spastic contractions and to retreat to a relaxed baseline whenever spasticity occurs. To reduce hyperadduction of the vocal folds, the patient starts with a relaxed, breathy sigh of short duration, proceeds to short words beginning with /h/, then to open-mouth vowels, and then to a nasal consonant or continuant. Plosives and affricates should be avoided because of the excessive pressure and musculature movement involved. Murry (1984) suggested the use of nasal and liquid sounds to help "defuse" the explosive (strained-strangled) phonatory characteristics of Friedreich's ataxia. Duffy (1995) noted that laryngeal massage may help strained-strangled voices.

Duffy (1995) reviewed the management of the pseudobulbar effect (pathologic crying and laughing), which occurs more frequently in spastic dysarthria than in other types of dysarthria. Drug therapy and the modification of head turning that precedes crying were successful in some cases. This author remembers working with a dysarthric patient who exhibited pseudobulbar crying on almost every utterance. Therapy that included overall relaxation and prolonged pausing on a word-to-word basis seemed to help this patient.

Breathiness

The problem of breathiness results from insufficient glottal closure. Therefore, a main approach to therapy attempts to close the glottis during phonation. Some suggestions follow:

1. Coughing, clearing the throat, and counting in a hard manner.

2. The previously described pushing exercises (pulling apart interlocked fingers while saying "ee" or "oo").

3. Another technique based upon the pushing technique is the glottal attack using a phoneme. In this instance, the patient is taught to start hard contact phonation with a

vowel or diphthong (/ah, ay, ee, aw, oh, oo/). This manner of initiating phonation is then applied to the production of words, phrases, and sentences.

At first, with the pushing or glottal attack method, the patient may produce a string of vowels or diphthongs with half fully phonated and the others not; or a single word may be half breathy and half normal; or a group of words, sentences, and paragraphs may be half and half. The back and forth nature of clear or breathy voice can go on for a number of sessions. Eventually, if successful, all of the patient's output will be fully phonated.

4. In cases of unilateral vocal fold paralysis, teflon and silicon injections (Hammarberg et al., 1984; Reich & Lerman, 1978) have been used to bolster or increase the size of the paralyzed fold. When the paralyzed fold is brought closer to the midline, better vocal fold vibration is frequently possible. The use of collagen injections (Duffy, 1995) may be recommended for the same purpose as teflon. Collagen may be preferable because it is structurally similar to the natural collagen in the vocal folds and is subject to only limited absorption.

Prosody Impairment

Prosody, which involves intonation and rate, can be inferior in the dysarthric speaker, as compared to normal speakers (see LeDorze, Ouellet, & Ryalls, 1994). Ziegler, Hartmann, and Hoople (1993) found that syllabic timing was related to severity and intelligibility in dysarthric speakers. Frequently, impairments in prosody can be alleviated by varying the patient's pitch and controlling the rate.

Varying Pitch

Exercises can help the patient discriminate auditorily while directing the pitch higher and lower. This therapy can begin with utterance of simple notes of the scale, then expand the vocalization to individual words, phrases, and then to sentences. Although some of the following exercises have been suggested for dysarthria caused by Parkinson disease (American Parkinson Disease Association, n.d.), they can be employed with most dysarthric patients regardless of the cause.

In the following example, key words in a sentence are stressed to clarify and change meaning. After the clinician does it first, the patient says the same sentence several times, changing word stress and noting how the meaning may change.

I don't want that grey coat.	I don't want **that** grey coat.
I **don't** want that grey coat.	I don't want that **grey** coat.
I don't **want** that grey coat.	I don't want that grey **coat.**

In the next example, after the clinician does it first, the patient practices asking questions and giving answers. The patient raises and lowers his or her voice as indicated by the arrows.

Q. Are you going?↑	Q. Have you seen my sweater?↑
A. No, I'm not.↓	A. It's in the closet.↓
Q. Do you know her?↑	Q. Can you help her?↑
A. I think I do.↓	A. Yes, I can.↓
Q. Is it fixed?↑	Q. Do you think he needs it?↑
A. I guess it is.↓	A. Yes, he might.↓
Q. Can you talk clearly?↑	Q. Where is my book?↑
A. I am trying hard.↓	A. It's on the desk.↓

Controlling Rate

Most dysarthric patients will have a slower than normal speaking rate because of the physiologic limitations within the vocal tract. Some speakers will be so slow that it reduces intelligibility or interferes greatly with the naturalness of speech. One dysarthric patient complained about the impatience of people who hung up during a phone call. She was told to start her phone conversations by saying, "I speak slowly because of a condition. Please bear with me." This preface seemed to help in future phone conversations.

To achieve intelligibility, slowing down the dysarthric speaker's rate should bring about more control in the patient's attempts at consonant exaggeration. Yorkston, Beukelman, and Bell (1988) pointed out that naturalness of speaking should be preserved as much as possible; otherwise it will hinder intelligibility beyond any benefits achieved by slowing down the rate. The patient mentioned above is an example of how an extremely slow rate interfered with intelligibility.

Duffy (1995) described the techniques used in slowing down a dysarthric speaker's rate. They include the following:

1. delayed auditory feedback—the patient wears earphones, enabling him to hear his own feedback at a slower rate

2. pacing board—while speaking, the patient uses a board with raised portions at measured intervals; each raised portion can indicate when a syllable or word should be spoken

3. metronomes—each beat can be used to indicate a syllable or word marker

4. pointing on an alphabet board to the first letter of each word spoken—can increase the intelligibility of sounds, words, or sentences

5. flashing lights—each flash can signal a syllable or word marker

6. hand or finger tapping—each tap represents a syllable or word

7. rhythmic cueing—the clinician points to words in a rhythmic manner while the patient is reading a passage

8. visual feedback—this appears on a computer screen when the patient reads a passage

Loudness Impairment

Loudness can be varied through the use of breathing exercises. Specifically, the patient can be taught to be aware of the breathing cycle and then to control the exhalation phase during phonation. For example, the patient may initially be told to say "one-two" on one exhalation. Once this easy task is accomplished, the patient progresses to "three" and so on until he or she has gained the required control of both phonation and exhalation. From there, the patient can vary the loudness of his or her voice commensurate with the degree of breath control.

Intermittent loudness and inaudibility can be controlled by teaching the patient to slow down the rate of speech and speak syllable by syllable. Auditory training is essential to the development of self-monitoring skills for loudness levels. Because the respiratory process supplies the energy or force for speech, any impairment in this process should be properly evaluated and modified.

Most normal speakers pause for breath at appropriate phrase and idea points in an utterance. With many dysarthric speakers, the reduction in movement and control of respiratory muscles requires more frequent pauses between words. Several dysarthric patients with whom this author has worked had to take a breath before each word spoken. This may have been laborious, but for these patients it was the only way they could communicate in a relatively normal manner. Patients need to achieve a compromise between the usual pattern of word groupings and the number of words they can say clearly before pausing for breath. With the following set of exercises (American Parkinson Disease Association, n.d.), the clinician should always demonstrate what has to be done.

The clinician then instructs the patient to do the following:

1. To become aware of control over inhalation and exhalation, feel the movement of the stomach muscles as one breathes in and out (e.g., place hands on stomach; inhale slowly; exhale slowly; repeat several times; try to establish a regular pattern).

2. Coordinate the breath stream with saying vowel sounds. Inhale and then produce a continuous tone as one exhales. Hold each sound as long as the voice continuous to be strong. Do not extend the time if the voice trails off (e.g., inhale and then say "ah" on exhalation; rest; repeat with other vowels and diphthongs).

   Timing the length of each sound will provide the average time each sound can be maintained and indicate if there is improvement. Sustaining a strong steady tone for 7 to 8 seconds is an average range.

3. Counting is a good way to practice breath control (e.g., hold palm of hand about 5 inches away from mouth to feel the air stream as one speaks; count from 1 to 10, inhaling and exhaling after each number; try to say each number with a firm, strong tone). The same exercise can be done with individual alphabet letters. Build up to as many numbers or

alphabet letters as possible on one exhalation without fading. It is better to say one or two words clearly than to say four or five words that are unintelligible.

4. Practice breath control with short phrases. Inhale first and then say each word separately on exhalation (e.g., "read /a/ book, brush /your/ hair, walk /the/ dog, knife /and/ fork, gang /of/ men, change /the/ time, reach /the/ park, push /and/ pull, jump /for/ joy, lots /of/ fun").

5. Practice additional short phrases. Try to say the whole phrase on one exhalation (e.g., "can of soup, go to sleep, pot of gold, just for fun, cup of soup, pinch of salt, time to go, next in line, come for brunch, join the crowd").

6. Practice phrasing with short sentences. Pause between phrases where marked (e.g., "we need/more soup, it's time/for brunch, Meg broke/the plate, please get/my hat, Jack lost/the new book, turn right/at the light, bring the bag/to the yard, Pat can come/later on, Ted caught/a big fish, put my shirt/on the table").

7. Practice modulating voice from soft to loud. Say "ah" in a soft tone and gradually increase the loudness. Repeat several times. Inhale each time at start of exercise and stop when voice fades.

8. Practice short phrases using three levels of loudness for each phrase. Imagine talking to listeners in different settings, first to a listener sitting opposite, then to a listener across the room, then to a listener in another room. Read across, not down, with each of the following:

To a Listener Opposite (softly)	TO A LISTENER ACROSS THE ROOM (A LITTLE LOUDER)	TO A LISTENER IN ANOTHER ROOM (MUCH LOUDER)
I won't	I WON'T	I WON'T
you can't	YOU CAN'T	YOU CAN'T
don't try	DON'T TRY	DON'T TRY
sit down	SIT DOWN	SIT DOWN
stop here	STOP HERE	STOP HERE

don't rush	DON'T RUSH	**DON'T RUSH**
he's okay	HE'S OKAY	**HE'S OKAY**
keep still	KEEP STILL	**KEEP STILL**
so long	SO LONG	**SO LONG**

9. Practice short sentences, using the same procedure as in number 8 to practice three levels of loudness.

To a Listener Opposite (softly)	TO A LISTENER ACROSS THE ROOM (A LITTLE LOUDER)	**TO A LISTENER IN ANOTHER ROOM (MUCH LOUDER)**
Look, Bill's awake.	GO TO SLEEP.	**THE MAILMAN JUST CAME.**
Is that Mary?	BRING ME MY PEN.	**WHO WANTS PIE?**
I've got a nickel.	CLOSE THE BOOK.	**YOU HAVE A PHONE CALL.**

10. Say each of the following phrases twice in succession, as if repeating a command; on the second phrase, speak louder. Inhale before each phrase.

keep quiet	KEEP QUIET
don't go	DON'T GO
go slow	GO SLOW
be still	BE STILL
sit up	SIT UP
hurry out	HURRY OUT
look out	LOOK OUT
first down	FIRST DOWN
come back	COME BACK
move away	MOVE AWAY

For those dysarthric patients who need it, Duffy (1995) reviewed the factors for increasing respiratory support (producing consistent subglottal air pressure, postural adjustments) and for prosthetic assistance (abdominal binders or corsets, expiratory boards or paddles). McNamara (1983) noted that a biofeedback instrument with visual feedback improved vocal loudness in a dysarthric patient. Particularly for ataxic dysarthria, Murry (1984) suggested that loudness is rarely worked on alone. Proper phrasing and breathing, and multisyllabic words are used to control loudness.

Ramig (1995) outlined the Lee Silverman Voice Treatment Program for Parkinson disease. Much of that program centers around techniques for improving loudness, some of which have been described previously in this treatment section. Studying a single patient with Parkinson disease, Dromey, Ramig, and Johnson (1995) found that vocal intensity treatment not only helped to increase his vocal loudness, but also led to better articulation, which was not targeted in treatment.

Ramig, Countryman, Thompson, and Horii (1995) observed that intensive voice and respiration treatment, focusing on increased vocal fold adduction and respiration exercises, was more effective for improving vocal intensity in 45 Parkinson disease patients than was respiration treatment alone.

Analyzing the same 45 Parkinson disease patients, Ramig and Dromey (1996) found that the combination of increased vocal fold adduction and subglottal pressure is a key in generating posttreatment increases in vocal intensity in idiopathic Parkinson disease. Countryman, Hicks, Ramig, and Smith (1997) found that vocal fold adduction therapy increased vocal loudness, decreased supraglottic hyperadduction, and improved intonation and overall voice quality in an individual with Parkinson disease who had reduced vocal loudness and supraglottic hyperadduction.

Duffy (1995), Netsell (1994), and Rosenbek & LaPointe (1985) reviewed the instrumentation (biofeedback devices such as water manometers, air pressure transducers, etc.) and speech methods (postural adjustments, muscle strengthening, controlled exhalation, etc.) used in the diagnosis and treatment of respiratory problems.

Severe Dysarthria

For the severely dysarthric speaker, Kangas and Lloyd (1998), Owens and House (1984), Shane and Bashir (1980), and Silverman (1989) offered criteria for determining candidacy for an augmentative or alternative system. They included a consideration of cognitive, oral reflex, language, motor, intelligibility, emotional, chronological age, previous therapy, imitative, and environmental factors.

Kangas and Lloyd (1998), Shane and Sauer (1986), and Silverman (1989) reviewed the augmentative or alternative communication strategies that have been used with dysarthric patients. These include manual sign languages, gestural morse code, nonelectronic communication (or conversation boards), electronic communication systems, computerized devices, and Blissymbolics (electronic & nonelectronic).

In cases of severe velopharyngeal incompetency, a palatal lift may be used to aid in producing closure of that area. This prosthesis is attached to the teeth and is made in the shape of a bulb obturator, with a hard plastic shelf attached to the posterior section of the palatal portion. This shelf projects posteriorly under the soft palate and maintains the palate in an elevated position (see Hardy, Netsell, Schweiger, & Morris, 1969).

With the use of a palatal lift, there has been success in reducing hypernasality and nasal emission and in increasing the overall intelligibility of speech in dysarthric children (Kent & Netsell, 1978), in developmentally delayed children (Shaughnessy, Netsell, & Farrage, 1983), and in dysarthric adults (Brand, Matsko, & Avart, 1988; Netsell, 1995). Duffy (1995) noted the use of pharyngeal flap surgery as a means for managing velopharyngeal incompetence in dysarthric speakers, although the much preferred method is a palatal lift prosthesis.

Additional types, reviews of evaluation procedures, and speech methods used in the treatment of dysarthria can be found in Bellaire, Yorkston, and Beukelman (1986), Duffy (1995), LaPointe and Katz (1998), Rosenbek and LaPointe (1985), Simpson, Till, and Goff (1988), and Yorkston, Beukelman, and Honsinger (1989). Reviews of nonspeech communication can be found in Kangas and Lloyd (1998), Shane and Sauer (1986), and Silverman (1989).

The third goal of therapy is to encourage the patient and the caretaker(s) to continue the rehabilitative process outside of the clinical setting.

Carryover, or the ability to use the correction consistently in normal conversation, is achieved by making the patient aware of his or her error while speaking, and motivating him or her to practice. Some techniques used in achieving carryover are giving the patient a clear understanding of the problem; objectifying progress through tape recordings, graphs, and charts; giving assignments with practice; and enlisting the family's or caretaker's help.

For example, the patient can practice reading aloud lists of words, phrases, sentences, and paragraphs. One dysarthric patient who had articulation and projection problems was a former nonprofessional singer who had performed in churches, at family get-togethers, and just for fun. As a result of her interest in singing, she had a vast repertoire of popular music. After each lesson, her assignment was to choose two songs and to concentrate on the articulation and projection. We called this practice assignment with singing "Stump the Clinician," which she accomplished about 50% of the time.

Another dysarthric patient, a retired high school teacher, had mis-articulations and a weak, monotonous voice. She loved poetry, and her assignment was to pick out her favorite passages of poetry and recite them aloud. The instructions were to imagine auditioning for a radio program and to concentrate on the proper articulation, projection, and vocal variety. The point was that both patients practiced, which was the purpose. The suggestions listed here for achieving carryover may be applied, with adaptations, to the other speech problems described in this chapter and in Chapter 8.

Improving Comprehensibility

Yorkston, Strand, and Kennedy (1996) suggested some techniques for improving comprehensibility (listener understanding of speech in a communicative setting) between the dysarthric speaker and the listener.

What the *listener* can do to aid comprehensibility is

- know the general topic of the conversation (e.g., encourage the dysarthric speaker to let the listener know beforehand, through any means, what the theme will be);
- watch for turn-taking signs (e.g., look at verbal, gestural, and body language signs that the dysarthric patient shows when he or she wants to speak);
- give the speaker undivided attention;
- pick the right time and place for communication (e.g., not when the patient is tired or upset);
- look at the dysarthric speaker;

- avoid talking when not in the same room; and

- determine and use strategies for resolving communication breakdowns by the dysarthric speaker (e.g., repeating misunderstood words, rephrasing, verbal spelling, writing).

What the *dysarthric speaker* can do to aid comprehensibility is

- provide the listener with the context of the topic (e.g., through writing or spelling of the topic heading);

- avoid shifting topics abruptly;

- choose proper turn-taking signals (e.g., eye gaze, a breathing pattern, a body movement, a gesture, verbal interjection);

- get the listener's attention (e.g., saying listener's name);

- use predictable wording and sentences (e.g., avoid unusual idioms, slang, and longer, grammatically complicated sentences);

- accompany speech with simple gestures (e.g., use index finger to make a circle, use hand to indicate a traffic cop's stop signal);

- avoid extended talking when not in same room as listener (e.g., use a buzzer or bell to get listener's attention);

- have a handy back-up system in case of difficulty (e.g., alphabet boards, pencil and paper); and

- use the previously mentioned repair strategies for resolving communication breakdowns.

In light of the above suggestions, Garcia and Cannito (1996) found that when signal fidelity is poor, as with the severe, flaccid dysarthric speaker, differing combinations of signal-independent information (gestures, predictiveness of message content, relatedness of sentences to specific situational contexts, and prior familiarity with the speaker) may be employed to enhance listener understanding of the spoken message.

CHAPTER 8

Apraxia of Speech

Definition

Apraxia of speech (AOS) is an articulation and prosody disorder that results from impairment, due to brain damage, of the capacity to order the positioning of the speech musculature and the sequencing of muscle movements for volitional production of phonemes and sequences of phonemes. It is not accompanied by significant weakness, slowness, or incoordination of these same muscles in reflex and automatic acts (Darley, 1964; Johns & Darley, 1970).

Conceptual-Programming Level of Motor Organization for Speech

Apraxia of speech has been described by Darley et al. (1975) as a planning or programming disorder that fits into a five-stage, conceptual-programming level of motor organization for speech.

The *first stage* is conceptualization, involving a desire to do something and establishing a plan of action to carry out that desire (e.g., thinking about calling a friend on the phone). In this stage, cortical activity is probably bilateral and widespread, and if interfered with can result, for example, in a cognitive thought disorder called dementia.

The *second stage* is spatial-temporal (linguistic planning), involving language (e.g., planning what one will say on the phone). In this stage, cortical activity for linguistic processes is located in the left hemisphere for the great majority of people, and if interfered with, can result in aphasia.

The *third stage* is motor planning (programming), which is the bridge between the language formulation and the motor execution stage of the neuromuscular system (e.g., talking on the phone). This stage is responsible for connecting the inner language processes into the endless number of speech utterances. It has been surmised that about 100 different muscles, each containing about 100 motor units, are involved in speaking for 1 second.

If an individual averages about 14 phonemes per second, then there are 140,000 neuromuscular events for 1 second of speech. Because of the complexity and the almost instantaneous speed and timing of those movements needed for speech, it is postulated that these movements have been stored in the brain (preprogrammed), ready to be activated at a moment's notice.

The storage of these movements starts in early childhood, and their individual strength is determined by the frequency of usage over a lifetime of speaking. For example, this author has heard a majority of patients say, "He could never make up his *filthy* mind" instead of the correct version, "He could never make up his *flighty* mind," when reading aloud the phonetically balanced passage called "Arthur the Young Rat." Apparently, "filthy mind" has been used more often (strong storage) than "flighty mind" (weaker storage).

In this stage, brain activity for motor planning is located for the great majority of people in the left hemisphere, involving Broca's area and its connections to the language portions of the temporal and parietal lobes, primary motor cortex (frontal lobe), supplementary motor area (frontal lobe), somatosensory cortex (parietal lobe), supramarginal gyrus (parietal lobe), and insula. If this stage is interfered with, the result can be apraxia of speech.

The *fourth stage* is performance, which is the motor execution portion of the neuromuscular system involved in speaking (e.g., talking on the phone). The brain activity is bilateral and involves the direct and indirect activation pathways, the control circuits, the final common pathway, feedback from sensory pathways, and continuous commands from the motor speech programmer. If this stage is interfered with, it can result in dysarthria.

The *fifth stage* is feedback, which provides sensory information about ongoing and completed motor speech movements. The modification of presently occurring and future motor speech movements is based upon this sensory information (e.g., getting a shot of Novocaine and compensating for the numbness in your lip and/or tongue in order to speak). The brain activity may occur at the spinal and brain stem level, in the cerebellum, thalamus, basal ganglia, and cortex. If this stage is interfered with, the result can be dysarthria.

Symptoms

Apraxia of speech can affect timing, rate, or range of movement of the articulators, and selection of articulatory contact points along the vocal tract. Salient features include disturbed articulation (inconsistent trial-and-error misarticulations) and prosody (hesitations, slowness, groping, difficulty initiating speech, dysprosody) with pockets of correct speech. Most often, patients are aware of their errors and can become frustrated when they can't correct themselves. This disorder can resemble the oral expressive language behavior of the aphasic patient. For example, the phonemic groping of the apraxic patient can resemble the word-finding difficulty of the aphasic patient. Apraxia of speech can stand alone as a condition, coexist with aphasia, coexist with dysarthria, or coexist with aphasia and dysarthria.

Following is an example of an apraxia of speech patient repeating words, phrases, and sentences first spoken by the clinician (the author).

Clinician	Patient
snowman	Snugman-smug-snowman
gingerbread	gingerbed
impossibility	in-impossibility
Please sit down	Please sit down.
seventeen seventy-six	senerteen senerty-six-severteen seventy-six
Columbia Presbyterian Hospital	Columbia Pesbyterian Hostiple-Columbian Presyterian Hostiple
Methodist Episcopal Church	Methodiss Epusiple Church-Methodist Episical Church

Will you answer the telephone?	Will<u>ee</u> <u>ll</u>oo <u>l</u>ans<u>it</u> <u>l</u>uh telesone-Will<u>ee</u> <u>ll</u>oo lans<u>it</u> <u>l</u>uh tel<u>e</u>tone?
No ifs, ands, or buts	No i<u>ss</u> and or buts - No i<u>ts</u> and or buts
He lives in the third house from the corner.	He'<u>d</u> live<u>d</u> in the <u>t</u>ird _ouse <u>f</u>om <u>d</u>uh <u>t</u>orner.

The following studies describe the symptoms of apraxia of speech. Many of the studies cited come from the review by Darley (1982), supplemented by the other literature listed.

1. Articulatory errors increase as the complexity of motor adjustment required of the articulators increases.

A. Vowels evoke fewer errors than singleton consonants (Wertz, LaPointe, & Rosenbek, 1984). Odell, McNeil, Rosenbek, and Hunter (1991) found that no differences existed in number of errors between vowels and consonants among apraxia of speech speakers.

B. Of the singleton consonants, affricative and fricative phonemes evoke the most errors (Wertz et al., 1984).

C. Most difficult of all are consonant clusters (Burns & Canter, 1977; Deal & Darley, 1972; Dunlop & Marquardt, 1977; Johns & Darley, 1970; LaPointe & Johns, 1975; Shankweiler & Harris, 1966; Trost & Canter, 1974; Wertz et al., 1984).

D. Palatal and dental phonemes are significantly more susceptible to error than other phonemes classified according to place of articulation (LaPointe & Johns, 1975).

E. In manner of articulation, fricatives and affricatives are least retained (Klich, Ireland, & Weidner, 1979).

F. Repetition of a single consonant such as /puh/, /tuh/, or /kuh/ is ordinarily accomplished more easily than repetition of the sequence /puh-tuh-kuh/ (Rosenbek, Wertz, & Darley, 1973). On the latter task the patient is typically unable to maintain the correct sequence, even when he or she is repeatedly given a model to imitate.

G. Klich et al. (1979), Marquardt, Reinhart, and Peterson (1979), and Wolk (1986) noted that apraxic patients made a systematic effort to reduce the articulatory complexity in the production of consonants. Keller (1984) also found that apraxic subjects tended to reduce the proportion of phoneme sequences (e.g., consonant clusters and diphthongs) and to increase the proportion of single consonants and single vowels in their speech.

H. Wertz et al. (1984) noted that a given sound can be correct in one position in a word but incorrect in another. They also noted that the production of easier consonants in place of more difficult ones is highly variable.

2. Position of phoneme within the word has an effect on articulatory errors.

A. *Consonants.* Initial consonants tend to be misarticulated more often than consonants in other positions (Hecaen, 1972; Shankweiler & Harris, 1966; Trost & Canter, 1974). Burns and Canter (1977) found that five patients with conduction aphasia and five with Wernicke's aphasia (mostly with posterior lesions) made what the authors called "phonemic paraphasic errors" more frequently in the final than in the initial position of words.

However, Johns and Darley (1970) reported that no single position in the word emerged as characteristically more difficult. LaPointe and Johns (1975) found error percentages for initial, medial, and final positions to be nearly equal, and Dunlop and Marquardt (1977) found phonemic position unrelated to occurrence of error. Klich et al. (1979) found that more substitutions were made in the initial word position. Wertz et al. (1984) concluded that sound position in a word may or may not have an influence on whether it will be produced accurately. Odell, McNeil, Rosenbek, and Hunter (1990) found that in consonant production by apraxic speakers, most errors occured in the medial position of words.

B. *Vowels.* In a follow-up study, Odell et al. (1991) found that in vowel production by apraxic speakers, most errors occurred in the initial position of words.

3. On repeated readings of the same material, apraxic patients demonstrate a consistency effect, tending to make errors at the same

loci from trial to trial; they also demonstrate some adaptation effect, tending to make fewer errors in successive readings (Deal, 1974). The amount of reduction of errors is not great, varying from subject to subject.

4. Phonemes occurring with relatively high frequency in the language tend to be more accurately articulated than phonemes that occur less frequently (Trost & Canter, 1974; Wertz et al., 1984).

5. Numerous phonemic errors occur, including substitutions, omissions, additions, repetitions, and distortions, with a predominance of substitutions (Johns & Darley, 1970; LaPointe & Johns, 1975; LaPointe & Wertz, 1974; Trost, 1970; Wertz et al., 1984). Analysis of substitution errors made by apraxic patients, according to the system of distinctive features, indicates that the errors are variably related to the target sounds. In their review of the literature, Wertz et al. (1984) conclude that generally, "apraxic patients are in the ballpark, most of the time. One or two phonetic feature errors predominate" (pp. 53–57).

Wertz et al. (1984) further concluded that apraxic patients generally "make more substitutions of voiceless consonants for voiced ones rather than the opposite" (p. 57). However, Skenes and Trullinger (1988) found that apraxic speakers made more errors on voiced than on voiceless consonants in tasks involving repetition of consonant-vowel-consonant. Odell et al (1990) observed that distortion errors predominated in consonant production, and Odell et al. (1991) found that distortion errors predominated in the vowel production of apraxic speakers.

6. When errors made by apraxic patients are analyzed with regard to sequential aspects, three types of errors are observed: anticipatory (prepositioning), reiterative (postpositioning), and metathesis (the order of two phonemes being reversed) (LaPointe & Johns, 1975). Wertz et al. (1984) noted that some patients display all three kinds of errors, with the anticipatory most frequent. However, all types of errors did not abound.

7. Apraxic patients display a marked discrepancy between their relatively good performance on automatic and reactive speech productions and their relatively poor volitional-purposive speech performance. "Words and phrases highly organized by practice and usage tend to sound normal" (Schuell et al., 1964, p. 265). Such islands of fluent, well-articulated speech appear in conversation, punctuated by episodes of effortful, off-target groping (LaPointe & Wertz, 1974; Wertz et al., 1984).

8. Imitative responses tend to be characterized by more articulatory errors than spontaneous speech production. This holds true for single monosyllabic words as well as for material of greater length and complexity. Some patients display remarkably long latencies between the presentation of a stimulus word and their repetition of it (Schuell et al., 1964; Johns & Darley, 1970; Trost, 1970). On the other hand, Wertz et al. (1984) found imitation to be better than spontaneous speech.

9. Articulation errors increase as length of words increases (Deal & Darley, 1972; DiSimoni & Darley, 1977; Wertz et al., 1984). As the patient produces a series of words with increasing numbers of syllables (e.g., *door, doorknob, doorkeeper, dormitory*), more errors are noted in all longer words. Such errors typically occur in the syllable common to all of the words, not just in the added syllables (Johns & Darley, 1970).

Odell et al. (1990) found no difference in number of errors between consonant production of monosyllabic and polysyllabic words; Odell et al. (1991) found more errors in vowel production of monosyllabic than of polysyllabic words in apraxic speakers.

10. In oral reading of contextual material, articulatory errors do not occur at random; they are more frequent on words that carry linguistic or psychologic "weight" and that are more essential for communication (Deal & Darley, 1972; Hardison, Marquardt, & Peterson, 1977). The combination of word length and grammatical class is an especially important determinant of the loci of errors. The difficulty level of initial phonemes also has a particularly negative effect on articulatory accuracy, when combined with grammatical class.

Grammatical class alone has not been found to be significantly related to occurrence of error (Deal & Darley, 1972; Dunlop & Marquardt, 1977; Wertz et al., 1984). Strand & McNeil (1996) observed that their five apraxic speakers consistently produced longer vowel and between-word segment durations in sentence contexts than in word contexts. In general, when the complexity of a required response is increased, more errors occur. Any single characteristic may be insufficient to elicit error, but if characteristics are combined, their joint effect may be powerful enough to induce inaccuracies.

11. Correctness of articulation is influenced by mode of stimulus presentation (Johns & Darley, 1970; Trost & Canter, 1974). Patients tend to articulate more accurately when speech stimuli are presented by a visible examiner (auditory-visual mode) than when they are presented by tape recorder (auditory mode) or printed on a card (visual mode).

Wertz et al. (1984) noted that the influence of stimulus mode is highly variable and depends on the individual patient.

12. Johns and Darley (1970) found that attainment of the correct articulation target is facilitated more by repeated trials of a word than by increase in the number of stimulus presentations. Patients are more likely to be on target if they are given a model once and have three opportunities to imitate it, than if they are permitted a single trial or are given three presentations of a model but only one trial to imitate it. LaPointe and Horner (1976) and Warren (1977) concluded that apraxic patients were extremely variable in their ability to improve on repeated trials. Wertz et al. (1984) observed that the process of repeated trials to aid facilitation is highly variable and depends a good deal on the clinical process.

13. Accuracy of articulation in apraxic patients is not significantly influenced by a number of auditory, visual, and psychologic variables. For example, when patients perform a task under two conditions, one while observing themselves in the mirror and the other without such visual monitoring, the difference in the number of errors they produce is not statistically significant (Deal & Darley, 1972). Similarly, introduction of masking noise that prevents patients from hearing their own speech does not significantly alter the number of articulation errors they make (Deal & Darley, 1972; Wertz et al., 1984).

Neither is articulatory accuracy influenced by the instructional set created in the speaker (Deal & Darley, 1972; Wertz et al., 1984). Patients do equally well (or poorly) in reading passages whether told that the passage is extremely easy, that it is loaded with hard words and phonemes and is extremely difficult, or that the degree of difficulty is unknown. Finally, incidence of errors is not significantly influenced by imposing upon the patient's speech an external auditory rhythm (metronome) (Shane & Darley, 1978; Wertz et al., 1984).

14. Aronson (1990) noted that in apraxia of speech, the laryngeal-phonatory characteristics include the following: phonation varies from normal sounding to mutism; mutism and other attempts at phonation (e.g., whispered speech) are due to the inability to voluntarily produce phonation or respiration on command, or to imitate, although they can reflexively produce phonation (e.g., coughing) and respiration (e.g., for intake of oxygen and outgo of carbon dioxide). The physical appearance of the vocal folds is normal in structure and function.

Oral Apraxia

Apraxia of speech (AOS) and oral apraxia are related to each other in the sense that the speech musculature comes into play in both conditions. In apraxia of speech, the disturbance is in the speech musculature during speaking, whereas in oral apraxia the disturbance is in the speech musculature during nonspeaking activities.

Oral (also nonverbal or buccofacial) apraxia has been described as a difficulty in performing voluntary movements with the muscles of the lips, tongue, mandible, and larynx in nonspeech tasks (coughing, chewing, sucking, or swallowing), although automatic movements of the same muscles are preserved (Darley et al., 1975). Oral apraxia exists despite intact motor abilities, sensory function, and comprehension of the required task. Oral apraxia often accompanies AOS, but each of these disorders can also exist alone.

Benson and Ardila (1996) ascribed the sites of lesion that can produce oral apraxia (a form of ideomotor apraxia) as tissue damage (cortex or white matter pathways) involving (a) the supramarginal gyrus of the dominant parietal lobe, particularly the arcuate fasciculus; (b) the dominant hemisphere motor association cortex, or the white matter tissues underlying this region; and (c) the anterior corpus callosum and/or the pathways that traverse this interhemispheric connector.

Oral apraxia is evaluated by having the patient perform oral postures (after demonstration) such as mouth open, tongue out, show teeth, and pucker lips, and *oral movements* (after demonstration) such as tongue in and out, pucker and smile, blow air, whistle, and cough (DiSimoni, 1989).

Apraxia of Speech Versus Dysarthria

In an effort to clarify the distinction between dysarthria and apraxia of speech, Darley (1982), Darley et al. (1975), Duffy (1995), Halpern (1986), Wertz (1985), and Wertz et al. (1984) noted the following:

1. Dysarthria generally involves all speech levels (respiration, phonation, resonance, articulation, and prosody), whereas apraxia of

speech is primarily a disorder of articulation and prosody (may be caused by compensatory behaviors).

2. Usually dysarthria is characterized by distortion errors, whereas apraxia of speech is characterized by substitution errors.

3. Dysarthric errors are probably more consistent than apraxia of speech errors; however, mild dysarthria is probably less consistent than severe apraxia of speech.

4. Dysarthric speakers are relatively uninfluenced by the degree of automatic speech (counting, reciting days of the week or months of the year, etc.), speaking situation (spontaneous speech, reading aloud, imitation), or linguistic variables (word length, frequency of occurrence, meaningfulness). Speakers with apraxia of speech can do better with automatic speech as opposed to propositional speech; depending on the speaking situation, can show correct or incorrect responses; and can be influenced by linguistic variables.

5. In apraxia of speech, neurologic examination reveals no significant evidence of slowness, weakness, incoordination, or alteration of tone of the speech musculature as in dysarthria. Dysarthria does not occur with aphasia as often as does apraxia of speech.

6. In dysarthria, the presence of oral apraxia rarely occurs, whereas oral apraxia occurs more frequently with apraxia of speech.

7. Darley (1982) and Darley et al. (1975) further noted that at the onset of apraxia of speech, the patient may experience difficulty initiating phonation at will; once this difficulty passes, as it usually does in a few days, phonation and resonance are normal.

8. In dysarthria, the articulatory errors are characteristically errors of simplification (distortions and omissions). In apraxia of speech, there is a preponderance of errors that must be considered complications of speech (substitutions of other phonemes, additions of phonemes, substitutions of a consonant cluster for a single consonant, repetitions of phonemes, and prolongations of phonemes).

Dysarthric patients usually do not grope for correct articulatory positions, nor are they successful at immediate self-correction. In contrast, patients with apraxia of speech typically show trial-and-error groping and attempts at self-correction that are sometimes immediately successful. Speakers with dysarthria probably show less variable dysfluencies than speakers with apraxia of speech.

9. Rosenbek, Kent, and LaPointe (1984) noted that more distortion errors have crept into the symptomatology of apraxia of speech. In spite

of this, their clinical rule is that dysarthria is the most likely diagnosis if a patient has a high proportion of relatively consistent distortions. Apraxia of speech is the likely diagnosis if distortions are mixed with what sound like substitutions, especially if such errors are relatively inconsistent.

10. Ludlow, Connor, and Bassich (1987) found that dysarthric patients with Parkinson and Huntington's disease were not impaired in speech planning or initiation, but had poor control over speech events. Conversely, apraxia of speech is viewed as a planning or programming disorder that can involve initiation disturbances.

11. Odell et al. (1991) found that in vowel production,

> A. speakers with apraxia of speech and ataxic dysarthria both made more errors in initiating than in sequencing (usually apraxic patients make more such errors),
>
> B. there was no difference in number of errors between vowels and consonants (usually both groups make more errors on consonants),
>
> C. both apraxic and dysarthric groups made more distortion than substitution errors (usually dysarthric patients make more such errors),
>
> D. both apraxic and dysarthric groups made more errors in initial position than in other positions (usually apraxic patients make more such errors),
>
> E. both groups showed no difference in number of errors between monosyllabic and polysyllabic words (usually apraxic patients make more errors on polysyllabic words), and
>
> F. both groups made more errors on stressed syllables (usually apraxic patients make more errors on stressed syllables).

Apraxia of Speech Versus Phonemic or Literal Paraphasia

Table 8.1 lists features that differentiate apraxia of speech from phonemic or literal paraphasia. A major proportion of the material comes from the reviews by Duffy (1995) and Wertz, LaPointe, and Rosenbek (1984), supplemented by the other literature listed.

Table 8.1. Differences Between Apraxia of Speech and Phonemic or Literal Paraphasia

Apraxia of speech	Phonemic or literal paraphasia
A. Brain lesion usually in the frontal lobe of the left hemisphere.	A. Brain lesion usually in the temporal or parietal lobe of the left hemisphere.
B. CVA the predominant etiology.	B. CVA the predominant etiology.
C. A right hemiplegia is common.	C. Usually no hemiplegia is present.
D. Accompanying oral apraxia more common.	D. Accompanying oral apraxia less common.
E. If patient is also aphasic, it usually profiles as a Broca's aphasia. If patient is not aphasic, then performance in the other language modalities should be normal.	E. The language deficits typically profile as a conduction or Wernicke's aphasia. Performance in the other language modalities should be impaired.
F. Accompanying unilateral upper motor neuron dysarthria is more common.	F. Accompanying unilateral upper motor neuron dysarthria is less common.
G. Speech characteristics:	G. Speech characteristics:
1. a lower proportion of sequencing errors	1. a higher proportion of sequencing errors
2. a higher proportion of positioning (initiation) errors	2. a lower proportion of positioning (initiation) errors
3. more predictable substitutions of sounds (slightly off-target) and more lawful in relation to manner and place of articulation, and voiced and voiceless features	3. less predictable substitutions of sounds (more off-target) and less lawful in relation to manner and place of articulation, and voiced and voiceless features
4. more errors on sounds in the initial position	4. more errors on sounds in the medial and final positions
5. more nonfluent output, slow rate, and groping	5. more fluent output, normal rate, and nongroping
6. more distortion of supersegmentals (stress)	6. less distortion of supersegmentals (stress)
* Because of 5 & 6 prosody is more abnormal.	* Because of 5 & 6 prosody is less abnormal.
7. ability to repeat is equal or superior to spontaneous speech	7. ability to repeat is much worse than spontaneous speech
8. more recognition and more attempts to self-correct articulatory errors	8. less recognition and fewer attempts to self-correct articulatory errors
9. speech production therapy (articulation and prosody) most effective	9. language stimulation therapy (comprehension and expression) most effective

Additional Studies that Compare AOS, Dysarthric, Aphasic, and Normal Speakers

Square-Storer, Darley, and Sommers (1988) found that in nonspeech and speech processing skills, patients with *pure apraxia* performed as well as normal subjects, compared to aphasia patients. This finding lends support to the position that apraxia of speech is a disorder distinct from aphasia. Li and Williams (1990) tested patients with conduction, Broca's, and Wernicke's aphasia in their ability to repeat phrases and sentences. Subjects with conduction aphasia showed a greater number of phonemic attempts, word revisions, and word and phrase repetitions. Subjects with Broca's aphasia showed more phonemic errors and omissions. Patients with Wernicke's aphasia showed more unrelated words and jargon.

McNeil, Liss, Tseng, and Kent (1990) measured the effects of speech rate on the absolute and relative timing of the sentence production of AOS and conduction aphasia speakers. Their results showed that there was a phonetic-motoric component contributing to the speech patterns of both apraxia and conduction aphasia groups. McNeil, Weismer, Adams, and Mulligan (1990) found that speakers with dysarthria and apraxia showed greater instability on lip, jaw, and finger isometric force and static position control than did normal speakers and those with conduction aphasia. Speakers with conduction aphasia fall somewhere between speakers with dysarthria and apraxia and normal speakers.

Odell et al. (1991) concluded that conduction aphasia patients made more vowel substitutions than did apraxia of speech and ataxic dysarthria patients; conduction aphasia patients made more vowel errors on polysyllabic words than did apraxia of speech and ataxic dysarthria patients; conduction aphasia patients made more vowel errors in the final position than did apraxia of speech and ataxic dysarthria patients; and apraxia of speech and ataxic dysarthria patients made more vowel errors on stressed syllables than did conduction aphasia patients.

Seddoh et al. (1996) found that in speech timing measures, apraxia of speech patients had longer and more variable mean durations than did normal subjects. Although conduction aphasia patients had longer consonant-vowel and vowel durations, their productions were not more variable than those of normal subjects. The authors suggested that these findings support the view that apraxia of speech is a motor speech disorder, and that conduction aphasia is a phonological rather than a motoric condition.

Recently, Hough and Klich (1998) examined the timing relationships of EMG (electromyography) activity of lip muscles underlying vowel production in 2 normal individuals and 2 individuals with marked to severe apraxia of speech (AOS). They found that the relative amounts of time devoted to onset and offset of EMG activity for lip rounding are disorganized in AOS. Word length appeared to affect the timing of the onset and offset of muscle activity for both the normal and the AOS speakers. The authors suggested that in AOS, termination of EMG activity may be at least as disturbed as the initiation of EMG activity.

Additional Sources

Additional reviews and studies concerning concepts of apraxia of speech can be found in Ardila (1992), Duffy (1995), Hough and Klich (1998), Kent and Rosenbek (1983), Robin, Bean, and Folkins (1989), Rosenbek et al. (1984), Square and Martin (1994), and Wertz et al. (1984).

Etiology

The etiology for apraxia of speech is brain damage—most likely a unilateral lesion in the language dominant hemisphere, involving singly or in combination Broca's area (frontal lobe), the premotor cortex (frontal lobe), the supplementary motor area (frontal lobe), the somatosensory area (parietal lobe), the supramarginal gyrus (parietal lobe), or the insula (paralimbic area). The frontal lobe is involved most often, followed by the parietal lobe. Sometimes the temporal lobe or subcortical areas are implicated.

Duffy (1995) noted that the etiologies of 107 cases of apraxia of speech (primary speech pathology diagnosis) seen at the Mayo Clinic were as follows: vascular (58%), composed of single left hemisphere stroke (48%) and multiple strokes including left hemisphere (10%); degenerative (16%); traumatic (15%), composed of neurosurgical (13%) and closed head injury (2%); tumor, left hemisphere (6%); other (5%); and multiple causes (1%).

Diagnosis

Diagnostic procedures for determining apraxia of speech can involve (a) establishing background information, (b) giving a neurologic evaluation, (c) employing informal tests, and (d) employing formal tests.

Establishing Background Information and the Neurologic Evaluation

These procedures can be found at the beginning of the "Diagnosis" section of Chapter 3.

Informal Tests

In testing for apraxia of speech, the same alternating motion rate (AMR) and sequential motion rate (SMR) procedures can be used as described in the "Diagnosis" section of Chapter 7 (Dysarthria). The patient is asked to repeat sounds, syllables, words, and sentences after the examiner. For example, while looking for the previously described symptoms of apraxia of speech, the examiner asks the patient to do the following:

1. Prolong /ah/.

2. Prolong /ee/.

3. Prolong /oo/.

4. Repeat /puh/ rapidly.

5. Repeat /tuh/ rapidly.

6. Repeat /kuh/ rapidly.

7. Repeat /puh-tuh-kuh/ rapidly.

8. Repeat "snowman."

9. Repeat "gingerbread."

10. Repeat "impossibility."

11. Repeat "Please sit down."

12. Repeat "seventeen seventy-six."

13. Repeat "Columbia Presbyterian Hospital."

14. Repeat "Methodist Episcopal Church."

15. Repeat "Will you answer the telephone?"

16. Repeat "no ifs, ands, or buts."

17. Repeat "He lives in the third house from the corner."

Informal scoring can follow the guidelines proposed by Darley et al. (1975). The inability to begin any phonation at the laryngeal level may indicate apraxia of phonation, which is an early and transient problem. *Severe* AOS is indicated if the patient can produce only some sounds at the laryngeal level, or one or two words (often with correct articulation).

Sometimes the single word is used appropriately. For example, one patient who communicated in Spanish and English prior to his stroke was only able to produce the word "si" (yes), which he used appropriately. When a response of "si" was not called for, he could produce only incomprehensible language sounds as a response. At other times, the single word is used for all responses. One patient was able to produce only the word "time" or "time-time," which she used for every single oral response, regardless of what was called for.

Moderate AOS is indicated if the patient produces inconsistent trial-and-error substitutions, omissions, distortions, or additions of phonemes; stuttering-like hesitations and blocking on phonemes; or groping for sounds and words, difficulty in starting speaking, dysprosody, and pockets of correct articulation.

Mild AOS is indicated if the patient produces phonemes in a nearly normal manner in contextual speech, but shows apraxic phonemic errors when asked to produce more difficult multisyllabic words or those that include demanding consonant clusters.

Informal testing can also be accomplished by engaging the patient in normal conversation, or asking the patient to respond out loud to action pictures or to read aloud a phonetically balanced passage (e.g., grandfather passage). Particularly for these informal testing situations, the use of a tape recorder would be helpful. The clinician's knowledge of phonetic transcription is an asset too, especially when it is used to describe the highly unusual and inconsistent output of the AOS patient.

Formal Tests

The *Apraxia Battery for Adults* (Dabul, 1979) checks for apraxia of speech by having the patient produce a timed diadochokinetic task, repeat words of increasing length, name pictures within a specific time period, read out loud, produce automatic speech by counting, and engage in spontaneous speech. A quantified scoring method is incorporated in the test.

Wertz et al. (1984) described their *Motor Speech Evaluation* whose origin is spread throughout the literature. It is a screening tool that usually takes less than 20 minutes to administer. Scoring the test can be descriptive (e.g., *A* for apraxic productions, *P* for paraphasias, *D* for dysarthria, *U* for nondiagnostic errors, *O* for other errors, and *N* for normal responses). Scoring can also be multidimensional (e.g., utilizing the *Porch Index of Communicative Ability* [PICA, Porch, 1981] 16-point scale) or use narrow or broad phonetic transcription.

The tasks are traditional:

1. conversation

2. vowel prolongation

3. repetition of monosyllables /puh/, /tuh/, /kuh/

4. repetition of a sequence of monosyllables like /puh-tuh-kuh/

5. repetition of multisyllabic words

6. multiple trials with the same word

7. repetition of words that increase in length (e.g., *thick, thicken, thickening*)

8. repetition of monosyllabic words that contain the same initial and final sound (e.g., *mom, judge*)

9. repetition of sentences

10. counting forward and backward

11. picture description

12. repetition of sentences used volitionally to determine consistency of production

13. oral reading

Wertz et al. (1984) further discussed sound by position tests, the influence of stimulus modes, and procedures for scoring and determining severity. Wertz (1984) noted some of the difficulties in assessing apraxia of speech. He advocated using a comprehensive set of tasks sensitive enough to tap the ambiguous patient.

The *Comprehensive Apraxia Test* (CAT) (DiSimoni, 1989) checks the following:

1. 20 oral volitional movements (e.g., after demonstration, the patient has to pucker lips, move tongue side to side)

2. production of 33 phonemes (e.g., patient repeats "ee," "eye," "p")

3. four sets of alternate motion rate (e.g., "puh-puh-puh," "tuh-tuh-tuh")

4. production of 10 syllables in nonsense words (e.g., patient repeats /m-ee-m/) and 10 syllables in short, real words (e.g., patient repeats /m-ah-m/)

5. 13 utterances of increasing length (e.g., patient repeats "cowboy," "exercise," "instructor")

6. 80 nonsense items in contextual inference (e.g., patient repeats /toog/teep/).

This test uses a multidimensional scoring system based on errors of phonemes in manner and place of articulation, and in voiced and voiceless contexts.

Duffy (1995) described a set of tasks that combine portions of the *Motor Speech Evaluation* (Wertz et al., 1984) and unpublished Mayo Clinic tasks for assessing apraxia of speech. It includes a scoring code that may be used to signify apraxia of speech response, for example, *D* for distortion, *G* for groping, *S* for substitution, *SC* for attempt at articulatory self-correction, *DR* for delayed response, *AOE* for awareness of errors, *SE* for sequencing errors, *SR* for slow rate, and *SXS* for syllable-by-syllable production of multisyllabic words or phrases.

Another scoring method for assessing apraxia of speech is the numeric code adapted from the PICA (Porch, 1981), where 15 = correct in all respects, 14 = distorted, 13 = delayed, 10 = self-corrected articulatory error, 9 = correct after a stimulus repetition, 7 = error clearly related to target, 6 = error unrelated to target, 5 = rejection or stated inability to respond, 4 = unintelligible but differentiated from other responses, 3 = unintelligible and relatively undifferentiated from other responses.

Duffy (1995) further suggested the use of broad or narrow transcription after the patient repeats vowels, diphthongs, consonants, words, words of increasing length (*cat, catnip, catapult, catastrophe*), the same word three times, and sentences. The patient is also asked to do the following: repeat /puh, puh, puh . . ./, /tuh, tuh, tuh . . ./, /kuh, kuh, kuh . . ./, and /puh, tuh, kuh . . ./ as fast and as steadily as possible; count from 1 to 10; and say the days of the week. As the patient sings "Happy Birthday," "Jingle Bells," or another familiar tune, the examiner makes note of how well the tune is carried and how adequate the articulation is. The examination also describes the patient's abilities in conversation, narrative speech, and reading aloud.

Therapy

The first goal of therapy is to inform the patient and the caretaker(s) about the nature and the consequences of the disorder.

The patient with apraxia of speech has a motor speech problem that involves problems with articulation, prosody, and fluency, in any combination. Thinking abilities are normal or near normal, and language should be intact. If aphasia is present, as it often is, then language will be impaired.

Prognosis

Rosenbek (1984) and Wertz et al. (1984) noted that particular patients with apraxia of speech present symptoms that warrant a favorable prognosis. These patients have the following characteristics: are less than 1 month post-onset, suffered a small lesion confined to Broca's area, have minimal coexisting aphasia, do not display significant oral or nonverbal apraxia, are in good health, and have the stamina for intensive treatment.

In addition, the following combination of factors enhance the prognosis for improved speech: education, counseling, and drill, the patient's ability to learn and to generalize, and the patient's willingness to practice. The authors noted that untreated apraxia patients do not reach the same competence as do those who are treated. Thus, the prognosis for functional recovery is poor without treatment, fair with treatment for the severe patient, and good with treatment for the moderate to mild patient.

The second goal of therapy is to provide the appropriate treatment approaches and techniques.

Efficacy of Therapy for Apraxia of Speech

Duffy (1995) noted that efficacy of treatment studies for apraxia of speech consist primarily of case reports and single-subject design studies. These studies indicate that a number of approaches and techniques can be effective in treating apraxia of speech, particularly if aphasia is absent or not outstanding. Principles of motor learning that involve drill, self-learning and instruction, feedback, specificity of training, consistent and variable practice, and speed-accuracy trade-off tasks are important in treatment.

Several specific programs of treatment (described later in this chapter) have been identified as effective. They include the following: the eight-step continuum for treating apraxia of speech, prompts for restructuring oral muscular phonetic targets, melodic intonation therapy, multiple input phoneme therapy, voluntary control of involuntary utterances, and a number of specific techniques not tied to any one program but associated with many of them (e.g., phonetic derivation, phonetic placement, minimal contrasts). As Duffy (1995) and Wambaugh and Doyle (1994), cited by Wambaugh, Kalinyak-Flisger, West, and Doyle (1998) pointed out in their reviews, more efficacy of treatment studies are needed that compare therapy programs and techniques with one another.

General Principles

As mentioned in the discussion of therapy for dysarthria, the general principles that underlie therapy for the motor speech disorders (Darley et al., 1975) are applicable here. Wertz et al. (1984) pointed out that therapy for apraxia of speech should concentrate on the disordered articulation and therefore differ from the language stimulation and auditory and visual processing therapies appropriate to the aphasias or the dysarthrias, where multiple problems due to paralysis exist (e.g., mobility exercises for a weak musculature would be appropriate for many dysarthria patients, but is not called for in apraxia of speech).

In general, a variety of phonetic conditions affect articulatory accuracy of the AOS patient in fairly predictable ways. These phonetic conditions are as follows: consonants produce more errors than vowels; consonant clusters produce more errors than singletons; within singletons, affricates and fricatives produce the most errors; substitution errors are perceived more than distortions, omissions, additions, and repetitions, and these substitutions are complications rather than simplifications of the target phoneme.

Duffy (1995) noted that with substitutions, most errors are in place of articulation, followed by manner of articulation, then by the voiced-voiceless division, and finally by the oral-nasal division, which had the least errors. Within place of articulation, most errors occur on palatal and dental phonemes; bilabials and lingua-alveolar phonemes are least in error (Duffy, 1995). Within manner of articulation, affricates and fricatives produce the most errors. In addition, initial consonant or vowel in a word produce the most errors, performance is better on automatic speech than on nonautomatic speech, more errors occur on words that have linguistic or psychological weight, and real words are easier than nonsense words.

Additional factors are distance between successive phonemes, where likelihood of error increases as distance between successive points of articulation within an utterance increases; word length, where errors increase as words increase in length; and word frequency, where errors occur more readily on rare than on common words. Trost and Canter (1974) found that phonemes with relatively high frequency tend to be more accurately articulated than those that occur less frequently. Therapeutic principles derived from the phonetic conditions described above should be considered when beginning therapy.

Articulatory accuracy in apraxia of speech is influenced by mode of stimulus (Johns & Darley, 1970; Trost & Canter, 1974). Johns and Darley (1970) found that auditory-visual stimulation is better than auditory or visual stimulation alone—visual in this instance referring to watching the clinician as he or she speaks. However, LaPointe and Horner (1976) observed no differences in correct production among single and combined modes of stimulation. Deal and Darley (1972) found that apraxia patients do not achieve greater phonemic accuracy if they are allowed to monitor their own speech in a mirror.

Auditory training does not necessarily precede production when instituting therapy. The apraxia patient who is either purely or only mildly aphasic can show auditory perception difficulties, as Aten, Johns, and Darley (1971) demonstrated, or can have little or no auditory perception problems, as Square (1981) showed. Nor does therapy necessarily employ a motokinesthetic approach (manual manipulation of the articulators for correct production) when deficits in oral sensation and perception have been demonstrated (Rosenbek, Wertz, & Darley, 1973). Deutsch (1981) found that oral form identification deficits are not causally related to motor speech programming problems.

Therapy does emphasize the auditory and visual modalities, especially the visual, because these clinically appear to be the most potent in guiding the articulators. Although it has not been experimentally confirmed as yet, it appears that establishing or strengthening "visual memory" is most important to therapeutic success with the apraxia patient. The phonetic placement method of describing the correct manner and place of articulation and the correct voiced and voiceless components of phoneme production is useful.

In his review, Duffy (1995) mentioned that in AOS, abnormalities occur in rate (e.g., slower than normal), prosody (e.g., equal stress on all syllables within a word), and fluency (e.g., groping for and/or repeating sounds and syllables).

Specific Phonemic Therapy Techniques

An Eight-Step Continuum for Treatment

Using the general principles mentioned above, Rosenbek, Lemme, Ahern, Harris, and Wertz (1973) advocate an eight-step integral stimulation ("Watch me and listen to me") method as an approach to therapy with apraxia patients. The eight steps are presented below using *bat* (as in *baseball bat*) as an example of a target word.

1. After integral stimulation by the clinician, the patient and the clinician say "bat" at the same time.

2. There is integral stimulation by the clinician, then after a delay the clinician mimes or repeats "bat" soundlessly (visual cue only), and the patient tries to say it out loud.

3. There is integral stimulation by the clinician, and after a delay the patient tries to say "bat" without any visual cue.

4. There is integral stimulation by the clinician, and after a delay the patient tries to say "bat" several times consecutively without any intervening auditory or visual cues.

5. The patient reads out loud the written or printed word *bat*.

6. The patient sees the written or printed word *bat*, reads it silently, and then says it out loud after the word is removed.

7. The imitative model is abandoned, and the clinician provides conditions so that the target utterance can be used volitionally as the correct response to a question (e.g., clinician says, "What do we hit a baseball with?" and patient attempts the word "bat").

8. The patient provides the appropriate response in a role playing situation (e.g., a mock ball game; clinician says, "You're at the plate with a _____" or "You're up next and swinging a _____").

Rosenbek, Lemme, et al. (1973) noted that the above steps can be employed on the syllable, word, phrase, or sentence level, and that patients need not go through all of the steps, especially those that are quite difficult. In addition, if integral stimulation does not work, other methods should be used (e.g., phonetic placement and phonetic derivation, which are described later). In a later study, Deal and Florance (1978) presented several successful cases that used a modified version of the eight-step continuum program.

Dabul and Bollier
Dabul and Bollier (1976) observed that apraxia patients' most characteristic problem is the sequencing of speech sounds. To improve this

condition they advocated the following sequential steps:

1. mastery of individual consonant phonemes
2. rapid repetition of each mastered consonant plus the vowel /ah/
3. build-up of sounds into syllables using CV, CV combinations, such as /fah, tah/, and CVC combinations such as /pahp/
4. after acquisition of a solid, basic "vocabulary" of articulatory positions, the patient attempts a difficult word by saying each phoneme in isolation and then blending the separate productions into syllables and words

Dabul and Bollier (1976) advocated the use of nonmeaningful syllable combinations in order to focus the patient's attention on the necessary phoneme sequencing and away from the decision of whether movements were voluntary or automatic. They found that mastery of volitional control over nonmeaningful syllable combinations leads to improved articulation of meaningful words. However, Kahn, Stannard, and Skinner (1998), Rosenbek (1984), and Wertz et al. (1984) favored the use of meaningful stimuli because of clinical success.

Melodic Intonation Therapy
Sparks and Holland (1976) reported success in using melodic intonation therapy (MIT) with nonfluent patients who exhibited relatively good auditory comprehension, frequent phonemic errors, and poor repetition skill. The intoned pattern is based on one of several speech prosody patterns that are reasonable choices for a given sentence, depending on the inference intended. The three elements are the melodic line, the rhythm, and points of stress. Through a gradual progression of carefully intoned sentences and phonemes, the patient is guided to normal prosody to aid speech return. A full discussion of this form of therapy can be found in Sparks and Deck (1994).

Rhythm Techniques
Rosenbek, Hansen, Baughman, and Lemme (1974) and Yoss and Darley (1974) found that various rhythmic techniques can facilitate the increase of articulatory accuracy. However, Shane and Darley (1978) found that auditory rhythmic stimulation (metronome) did not significantly im-

prove articulatory accuracy. Keith and Aronson (1975) described the use of singing as a form of apraxia of speech therapy.

Phonetic Derivation and Phonetic Placement

Rosenbek (1985) advocated using the phonetic derivation method, whereby target sounds are derived from intact nonspeech or speech gestures. For example, biting the lower lip produces /f, v/, puckering the lips produces /oo, oh, aw, w/, smiling produces /ee, eh/, yawning produces /ah, uh/, and wiping one's mouth produces /m, p, b/. The phonetic placement method of describing the correct manner and place of articulation, and the correct voiced and voiceless components of target phoneme production uses both visual and verbal instruction.

Prompts for Restructuring Oral Musculature Phonetic Targets

Another approach is PROMPT (Square-Storer & Hayden, 1989), which stands for prompts for restructuring oral musculature phonetic targets. This approach stresses the patient's kinesthetic awareness of speech movements or their prevention. The clinician provides tactile cues to various portions of the patient's vocal tract (e.g., touching patient's nose for a nasal sound or the lips for a bilabial sound, with the length of the touch determining the length of time the sound should be held). Once this heightened kinesthetic awareness is established, combinations of visual, auditory, and tactile input are used for the production of sounds, words, and short phrases.

Multiple Input Phoneme Therapy

Stevens (1989) described an approach called multiple input phoneme therapy (MIPT). Geared for severe apraxia patients, this approach takes the involuntary verbal stereotypes and tries to bring them under voluntary control. First the clinician repeats the stereotypic utterance, then has the patient repeat along with the clinician, and then both of them tap simultaneously along with the utterance. The initial phoneme of the utterance is stressed, and gradually the clinician's voice fades away until he or she is only mouthing the word(s) while the patient continues saying them. Other words beginning with that same phoneme are introduced, eventually leading to all phonemes, phrases, and short sentences. If all prior steps are successful, the repetitions are faded and patient responses are evoked, for example, by naming of pictures or reading cues.

Voluntary Control of Involuntary Utterances

Helm & Baresi (1980) developed the voluntary control of involuntary utterances (VCIU) for use with apraxia and aphasia patients. In this approach, the clinician writes down any real word the patient says in any speaking context. The clinician writes these words individually on cards for the patient to read aloud. If another real word is substituted for the target word, then the target word is scrapped and the substituted word is kept for future use as a target word.

Short, frequently used, easy initial phoneme, and emotion-laden words are suggested for building up a vocabulary. After the patient can read this vocabulary aloud, the next step would be having the patient name pictures or engage in controlled conversation that employs those words. All the while, any new words are added to the vocabulary.

Minimal Contrasts

The use of minimal contrasts in single words (e.g., "tea–key"), phrases. (e.g., "tan–coat"), and sentences (e.g., "Ted can tell Kay about the two cars") can be used to bolster each individual consonant and to differentiate between consonants that are close. Cognates are pairs of consonants that are alike in manner and place of articulation but differ in the voiced-voiceless category. Words beginning with cognate pairs (e.g., "pat–bat, to–do, fan–van, sue–zoo, Kay–gay") can also be used in contrast drills. Keith and Thomas (1989) provided practice materials for the vowels, diphthongs, and consonants for contrast purposes.

Recently, Wambaugh et al. (1998) studied the effects of a treatment for sound errors in three speakers with chronic apraxia of speech and aphasia. Treatment combined the use of minimal contrast pairs with traditional sound production training techniques such as integral stimulation and articulatory placement cueing, and was applied sequentially to sounds that were consistently in error before training. Results indicated increased correct sound productions for all speakers in trained and untrained words.

Traditional Therapy for the Patient with Severe Apraxia of Speech

To initiate phonation, the clinician (with the use of a mirror) should produce the sound /ah/ and have the patient watch and listen and then imitate. If the patient is unable to imitate the sound, the clinician should place the patient's hand on his or her larynx while he or she is attempting to phonate. Sometimes it may be necessary for the clinician to manually open the patient's mouth and shape his or her lips. This procedure should be repeated numerous times. The auditory stimulation by the clinician and from the patient's own auditory feedback system, plus the tactile stimulation of holding the larynx should facilitate controlled production. Some severely involved patients may have to work on oromotor control to achieve any sort of sound.

Dworkin (1991) and Dworkin, Abkarian, and Johns (1988) described a number of nonspeech oromotor exercises for the lips, tongue, jaw, and respiratory system. Aronson (1990) recommended that establishing response hierarchies by going from a reflective sound such as a cough, clearing the throat, a moan, a grunt, a laugh, a sigh, or humming a tune, can facilitate the production of a volitional /ah/ sound. Volitional sound production can also be augmented by having the patient shape his or her lips with his or her own fingers. Duffy (1995) suggested pairing a highly used symbolic gesture with its associated sound or word (e.g., placing the index finger to the lips to say "sh," or blowing out a match to form vowel sounds).

Once the patient becomes successful in producing a volitional /ah/ sound, the characteristics of pitch, duration, and loudness become the goals of intervention. Subsequently, other vowel sounds (e.g., /ee, oo, oh/) can be worked on in the same manner. According to Darley et al. (1975), singing and completing automatic phrases (e.g., "a cup of _____," "grass is _____") can also be useful techniques for initiating phonation. They further suggested the use of everyday expressions such as "Hello," "How are you," "Thank you," and "Goodbye" and the use of overlearned material such as the Lord's Prayer, the Pledge of Allegiance, the 23rd psalm, nursery rhymes, and TV advertising jingles as means of eliciting full speech activities.

DiSimoni (1989) reviewed the use of augmentative or alternative systems that may be used with severely involved apraxia patients, either to augment or supplant the use of oral communication. These approaches include communication boards, mechanical communication systems, finger spelling, sign language, pantomine and gesture, writing, and picture drawing. Kangas and Lloyd (1998), Shane and Sauer (1986), and Silverman (1989) offered additional reviews of augmentative or alternative systems that can be used with the patient with severe apraxia of speech.

Traditional Therapy for the Patient
with Moderate and Mild Apraxia of Speech

Taking into account the previously described phonetic conditions that affect articulatory accuracy, additional phonemic therapy techniques involve working on individual vowels in the manner described under the "Traditional Therapy for the Patient with Severe Apraxia of Speech" section. When the patient has the vowel sounds (e.g., /ee, oo, oh/) at his or her command, the production of consonants can become the focus of therapeutic activity. For example, the /m/ sound, which is easily seen, might be a suitable consonant with which to begin therapy. The clinician produces the /m/ sound and then has the patient close his or her lips. If the patient is unable to perform this task, he or she should then be directed to imitate the clinician in closing and shaping the lips with his or her fingers. With the lips closed, the patient makes a humming sound.

Sometimes the patient will feel the clinician's larynx while the clinician produces this sound. The patient is encouraged to hum a familiar melody and receives feedback from the clinician concerning its correctness. The patient then reproduces the /m/ sound and subsequently changes his or her mouth position by opening his or her lips. This change in mouth position is used to overcome patient fear of being unable to produce a particular articulatory posture again. Thus, the clinician works on changing from /m/ to open mouth posture, or from /m/ to a vowel that is already in the patient's phonemic repertoire.

Once the /m/ can be produced in isolation, it can be used in the initial position with the vowels that were learned (e.g., /mah, moo, mee, moh/). If other vowels are developed spontaneously or in response to therapy, they can also be used. Next, /m/ is produced in the final position in one-syllable words (e.g., "am, I'm, arm"), two-syllable words (e.g., "mama, memo"), and then in word lists with /m/ in all positions (e.g., "madam, omen").

From there one can proceed to simple phrases (e.g., "my man, my mama, my money"), to longer phrases (e.g., "miles from Montana, music man, made men are mean"), and to sentences (e.g., "The mailman will get the mail. A memo was sent to the milkman. The marmalade came from Memphis"). This can be followed by working on differentiating similar sounding words with /m/ in the initial position (e.g., "man–pan, mail–pail, make–bake, mat–bat"), /m/ in the final position (e.g., "come–cub, dumb–dub"), and progressively longer words ("measure–measured–measurable, mean–meaning–meaning-ful"). More examples of progressively longer words can be found in Keith and Thomas (1989).

Patients with mild apraxia of speech can now forego many of the imitative tasks that were presented in the earlier forms of therapy. With self-monitoring skills (e.g., slowing down their rate of speaking), they can attempt full conversational activities. For examples of tasks that range from the formulation of simple sentences (e.g., clinician says, "What barks"? and patient answers using a sentence) to explaining the meaning of metaphors (e.g., "She's the apple of his eye") and similes (e.g., "happy as a clam"), see therapy suggestions OED 7 through OED 11 in the "Therapy" section of Chapter 3.

Facilitators in Apraxia of Speech Therapy

DiSimoni (1989) reviewed the facilitators in apraxia of speech therapy that have proven successful. They include the following:

1. procedures that pace the patient—metronomes, palilalia board, walk and talk, manual gesture for each word or sylla-ble, finger tapping reading aloud using a blind (usually a 3" × 5" card with a rectangular hole in it, placed over copy to be read so that only one word at a time is visible), pointing to words while reading, stressing underlined words, stressing different colored words, reading with print upside down or sideways, visualizing each word, visualizing a geometric figure, visualizing the first letter of each word

2. procedures that relax the patient—biofeedback, progressive relaxation

3. other procedures—standing while speaking phonemic prompts, hypnosis

Additional reviews and therapeutic techniques for apraxia of speech have been described by Darley et al. (1975), DiSimoni (1989), Duffy (1995), Dworkin (1991), Dworkin, Abkarian, and Johns (1988), Hough and Klich (1998), LaPointe and Katz (1998), Rosenbek, Kent, and LaPointe (1984), Square & Martin (1994), and Wertz et al. (1984).

The third goal of therapy is to encourage the patient and the caretaker(s) to continue the rehabilitative process outside of the clinical setting.

The ability to achieve carryover for the patient with apraxia of speech would follow guidelines similar to those mentioned for the patient with dysarthria (see Chapter 7). For example, this author remembers a patient with apraxia of speech who also had mild aphasia. He was a retired chemist who, along with thousands of other professionals, worked on the making of the first atomic bomb during World War II (the Manhattan Project). His assignment was to select, from books already in his possession, material relating to the Manhattan Project, rehearse it with his wife at home, and then present it orally to this author during the therapy session. In this way, he was practicing with his wife's help, away from the clinical setting, to help overcome his articulation and prosody problems resulting from the apraxia of speech and his word-finding difficulty caused by the aphasia.

To boot, this author learned a great deal from this erudite gentleman in the process of the assignment. For example, the patient mentioned that although he sensed that his specific area of chemistry was making a contribution to something of major importance, he did not know the nature of the finished product. That he learned via a memo circulated after the A-bomb was dropped on Hiroshima. In this way, the Manhattan Project, with thousands of people involved, was able to maintain its secrecy and prevent leaks. To the end, only a handful of people knew its ultimate goal. Throughout this entire narrative, the patient maintained a consistent and considerable improvement in articulation, prosody, and word-finding.

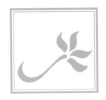

References

Abeysinghe, S., Bayles, K., & Trosset, M. (1990). Semantic memory deterioration in Alzheimer's subjects: Evidence from word association, definition, and associate ranking tasks. *Journal of Speech and Hearing Research, 33,* 574–582.

Ackerman, H., Hertrich, L., & Scharf, G. (1995). Kinemic analysis of lower lip movements in ataxic dysarthria. *Journal of Speech and Hearing Research, 38,* 1252–1259.

Adamovich, B. (1992). The role of the speech–language pathologist in the evaluation and treatment of adolescents and adults with traumatic brain injury. *Neurophysiology and neurogenic speech and language disorders, 2*(1). [Special Interest Division Newsletter; Rockville, MD: American Speech-Language-Hearing Association].

Adamovich, B., & Brooks, R. (1981). A diagnostic protocol to assess the communication deficits in patients with right hemisphere damage. In R. Brookshire (Ed.), *Clinical aphasiology conference proceedings* (pp. 244–253). Minneapolis, MN: BRK.

Adamovich, B., & Henderson, J. (1992). *Scales of Cognitive Ability for Traumatic Brain Injury (SCATBI).* Austin, TX: PRO-ED.

Alpert, M., Rosen, A., & Welkowitz, J. (1990). Interpersonal communication in the context of dementia. *Journal of Communication Disorders, 23,* 337–346.

American Parkinson Disease Association. (n.d.). *Speech problems and swallowing problems in Parkinson's disease.* New York: Author.

American Psychiatric Association. (1994). *Diagnostic and statistical manual of mental disorders* (4th ed.). Washington, DC: Author.

American Speech-Language-Hearing Association. (1991). Guidelines for speech-language pathologists serving persons with socio-communicative, and/or cognitive communicative impairments. *ASHA, 33*(Suppl. 5), 21–28.

American Speech-Language-Hearing Association. (1993). Definitions of communication disorders and variations. *ASHA, 35*(Suppl. 10), 40–41.

American Speech-Language-Hearing Association. (1994). *Functional assessment of communication skills for adults.* Bethesda, MD: Author.

Anderson, K., & Miller, P. (1986, November). *Clinical management of the right hemisphere damaged patient.* Short course presented at the meeting of the American Speech-Language-Hearing Association Convention, Detroit, MI.

Ansell, B. (1991). Slow-to-recover brain-injured patients: Rationale for treatment. *Journal of Speech and Hearing Research, 34,* 1017–1022.

Appell, J., Kertesz, A., & Fisman, M. (1982). A study of language functioning in Alzheimer's patients. *Brain & Language, 17,* 73–91.

Ardila, A. (1992). Phonological transformations in conduction aphasia. *Journal of Psycholinguistic Research, 21,* 473–484.

Aronson, A. (1990). *Clinical voice disorders.* New York: Thieme.

Aten, J. (1984). Treatment of spastic dysarthria. In W. Perkins (Ed.), *Dysarthria and apraxia* (pp. 69–77). New York: Thieme-Stratton.

Aten, J. (1994). Functional communication treatment. In R. Chapey (Ed.), *Language intervention strategies in adult aphasia* (pp. 292–303). Baltimore: Williams & Wilkins.

Aten, J., Johns, D., & Darley, F. (1971). Auditory perception of sequenced words in apraxia of speech. *Journal of Speech and Hearing Research, 14,* 131–143.

Au, R., Obler, L., & Albert, M. (1991). Language in aging and dementia. In M. Sarno (Ed.), *Acquired aphasia* (pp. 405–423). New York: Academic Press.

Baker, K., Ramig, L., Johnson, A., & Freed, C. (1997). Preliminary voice and speech analysis following fetal dopamine transplants in 5 individuals with Parkinson disease. *Journal of Speech-Language-Hearing Research, 40,* 615–626.

Barlow, S., & Abbs, J. (1983). Force transducers for the evaluation of labial, lingual, and mandibular motor impairments. *Journal of Speech and Hearing Research, 26,* 616–621.

Barlow, S., & Burton, M. (1990). Ramp-and-hold force control in the upper and lower lips: Developing new neuromotor assessment applications in traumatically brain injured adults. *Journal of Speech and Hearing Research, 33,* 660–675.

Barlow, S., Cole, K., & Abbs, J. (1983). A new head-mounted lip-jaw movement transduction system for the study of motor speech disorders. *Journal of Speech and Hearing Research, 26,* 283–288.

Basso, A., Capitani, E., & Vignolo, L. (1979). Influence of rehabilitation on language skills in aphasic patients: A controlled study. *Archives of Neurology, 36,* 190–196.

Bayles, K. (1982). Language function in senile dementia. *Brain & Language, 16,* 265–280.

Bayles, K. (1994). Management of neurogenic communication disorders associated with dementia. In R. Chapey (Ed.), *Language intervention strategies in adult aphasia* (pp. 535–545). Baltimore: Williams & Wilkins.

Bayles, K., & Boone, D. (1982). The potential of language tasks for identifying senile dementia. *Journal of Speech and Hearing Disorders, 47,* 210–217.

Bayles, K., Boone, D., Tomoeda, C., Slauson, T., & Kazniak, A. (1989). Differentiating Alzheimer's patients from the normal elderly and stroke patients with aphasia. *Journal of Speech and Hearing Disorders, 54,* 74–87.

Bayles, K., & Tomoeda, C. (1983). Confrontation naming impairment in dementia. *Brain & Language, 19,* 98–114.

Bayles, K., & Tomoeda, C. (1991). *Arizona Battery for Communication Disorders of Dementia.* Tucson, AZ: Canyonlands Publishing.

Bayles, K., & Tomoeda, C. (1996). Principles and techniques for managing the memory deficits of persons with mild to moderate dementia. *Neurophysiology and neurogenic speech and language disorders, 6*(3). [Special Interest Division Newsletter; Rockville, MD: American Speech-Language-Hearing Association].

Bayles, K., Tomoeda, C., & Caffrey, J. (1982). Language and dementia producing diseases. *Communication Disorders, 7,* 131–146.

Bayles, K., Tomoeda, C., Kazniak, A., Stern, L., & Eagans, K. (1985). Verbal perseveration of dementia patients. *Brain & Language, 25,* 102–116.

Bayles, K., Tomoeda, C., & Trosset, M. (1992). Relation of linguistic communication abilities of Alzheimer's patients to stage of disease. *Brain & Language, 42,* 454–472.

Bellaire, K., Yorkston, K., & Beukelman, D. (1986). Modification of breath patterning to increase naturalness of a mildly dysarthric speaker. *Journal of Communication Disorders, 19,* 271–280.

Benowitz, L., Moya, K., & Levine, D. (1990). Impaired verbal reasoning and constructional apraxia in subjects with right hemisphere damage. *Neuropsychologia, 28,* 231–241.

Benson, D. F. (1979). *Aphasia, alexia, agraphia.* New York: Churchill-Livingston, Inc.

Benson, D. F., & Ardila, A. (1996). *Aphasia: A clinical perspective.* New York: Oxford University Press.

Benton, A., & Hamsher, K. (1978). *Multilingual Aphasia Examination.* Iowa City, IA: Benton Lab. of Neuropsychology.

Berry, W. (1984). Treatment of hypokinetic dysarthria. In W. Perkins (Ed.), *Dysarthria and apraxia* (pp. 91–99). New York: Thieme-Stratton.

Berry, W., Darley, F., Aronson, A., & Goldstein, N. (1974). Dysarthria in Wilson's disease. *Journal of Speech and Hearing Research, 17,* 169–183.

Beukelman, D., & Yorkston, K. (1980). Influence of passage familiarity on intelligibility estimates of dysarthric speech. *Journal of Communication Disorders, 13,* 33–41.

Beukelman, D., Yorkston, K., & Waugh, P. (1980). Communication in severe aphasia: effectiveness of three instruction modalities. *Archives of Physical Medicine and Rehabilitation, 61,* 248–252.

Bloom, R., Borod, J., Obler, L., & Gerstman, L. (1992). Impact of emotional content on discourse production in patients with unilateral brain damage. *Brain and Language, 42,* 153–164.

Bloom, R., Borod, J., Obler, L., & Gerstman, L. (1993). Suppression and facilitation of pragmatic performance: Effects of emotional content on discourse following right and left brain damage. *Journal of Speech and Hearing Research, 36,* 1227–1235.

Boles, L. (1998). Conducting conversation: A case study using the spouse in aphasia treatment. *Neurophysiology and neurogenic speech and language disorders, 8*(3). [Special Interest Division Newsletter; Rockville, MD: American Speech-Language-Hearing Association].

Boller, F., Becker, J., Holland, A., Forbes, M., Hood, P., & McGonigle-Gibson, P. (1991). Predictions of decline in Alzheimer's disease. *Cortex, 27,* 9–17.

Boone, D. (1983). *The voice and voice therapy.* Englewood Cliffs, NJ: Prentice-Hall.

Borkowski, J., Benton, A., & Spreen, O. (1967). Word fluency and brain damage. *Neuropsychologia, 5,* 135–140.

Borod, J., Alpert, M., Brozgold, A., Martin, C., Welkowitz, J., Diller, L., Peselow, E., Angrist, B., & Lieberman, A. (1989). A preliminary comparison of flat affect schizophrenics and brain-damaged patients on measures of affective processing. *Journal of Communication Disorders, 22,* 93–104.

Bourgeois, M. (1991). Communication treatment for adults with dementia. *Journal of Speech and Hearing Research, 34,* 831–844.

Bourgeois, M. (1992). Evaluating memory wallets in conversation with persons with dementia. *Journal of Speech and Hearing Research, 35,* 1344–1357.

Bowles, N., Obler, L., & Albert, M. (1987). Naming errors in healthy aging and dementia of the Alzheimer type. *Cortex, 23*, 519–524.

Boyle, M., & Coelho, C. (1995). Application of semantic feature analysis as a treatment for aphasic dysnomia. *American Journal of Speech-Language Pathology, 4*, 94–99.

Bracy, C., & Drummond, S. (1993). Word retrieval in fluent and non-fluent dysphasia: Utilization of pictogram. *Journal of Communication Disorders, 26*, 113–128.

Brand, H., Matsko, T., & Avart, H. (1988). Speech prosthesis retention problems in dysarthria. *Archives of Physical Medicine and Rehabilitation, 69*, 213–214.

Brookshire, R. (1974). Differences in responding to auditory materials among aphasic patients. *Acta Symbolica, 5*, 1–18.

Brookshire, R. (1983). Subject description and generality of results in experiments with aphasic adults. *Journal of Speech and Hearing Disorders, 48*, 342–346.

Brookshire, R. (1994). Group studies of treatment for adults with aphasia: Efficacy, effectiveness, and believability. *Special Interests Division, Neurophysiology and neurogenic speech and language disorders, 4*(4). [Special Interest Division Newsletter; Rockville, MD: American Speech-Language-Hearing Association].

Brookshire, R. (1997). *An introduction to neurogenic communication disorders* (5th ed.). St. Louis, MO: Mosby Yearbook.

Brookshire, R., & Nicholas, L. (1997). *Discourse Comprehension Test.* Bloomington, MN: BRK Publishers.

Brown, J., & Perecman, E. (1986). Neurologic basis of language processing. In R. Chapey (Ed.), *Language intervention strategies in adult aphasia* (pp. 12–22). Baltimore: Williams & Wilkins.

Brownell, H., Potter, H., Bihrle, A., & Gardner, H. (1986). Inference deficits in right-brain damaged patients. *Brain & Language, 27*, 310–321.

Brownell, H., Simpson, T., Bihrle, A., Potter, H., & Gardner, H. (1990). Appreciation of metaphoric alternative word meanings by left and right brain-damaged patients. *Neuropsychologia, 28*, 375–383.

Bryan, K. (1989). *The Right Hemisphere Language Battery*. Leicester, England: Far Communications.

Burns, M., & Canter, G. (1977). Phonemic behavior of aphasic patients with posterior cerebral lesions. *Brain & Language, 4*, 492–507.

Burns, M., Halper, A., & Mogil, S. (1985). *Clinical management of right-hemisphere dysfunction*. Rockville, MD: Aspen Systems Corp.

Butfield, A., & Zangwill, O. (1946). Re-education in aphasia: A review of 70 cases. *Journal of Neurology, Neurosurgery, & Psychiatry, 9*, 75–79.

Caligiuri, M. (1989). The influence of speaking rate on articulatory hypokinesia in Parkinsonian dysarthria. *Brain & Language, 36*, 493–502.

Campbell, T., & Dollaghan, C. (1990). Expressive language recovery in severely brain-injured children and adolescents. *Journal of Speech and Hearing Disorders, 55*, 567–581.

Campbell, T., & Dollaghan, C. (1995). Speaking rate, articulatory speed, and linguistic processing in children and adolescents with severe traumatic brain injury. *Journal of Speech and Hearing Research, 38*, 864–875.

Canter, G., & Van Lancker, D. (1985). Disturbances of the temporal organization of speech following bilateral thalamic surgery in a patient with Parkinson's disease. *Journal of Communication Disorders, 18*, 329–349.

Cappa, S., Papagno, C., & Vallar, G. (1990). Language and verbal memory after right hemispheric stroke: A clinical-CT scan study. *Neuropsychologia, 28*, 503–509.

Cazzato, K. (1998). A case of functionally based rehabilitation following a mild traumatic brain injury. *Neurophysiology and neurogenic speech and language disorders, 8*(2). [Special Interest Division Newsletter; Rockville, MD: American Speech-Language-Hearing Association].

Chapey, R. (1994). Assessment of language disorders in adults. In R. Chapey (Ed.), *Language intervention strategies in adult aphasia* (pp. 80–120). Baltimore: Williams & Wilkins.

Chieffi, S., Carlomagno, S., Silveri, M., & Gainotti, G. (1989). The influence of semantic and perceptual factors in lexical comprehension in aphasic and right brain damaged patients. *Cortex, 25,* 591–598.

Code, C. (Ed.). (1989). *The characteristics of aphasia.* New York: Taylor & Francis.

Coelho, C. (1997). Cognitive-communicative disorders following traumatic brain injury. In C. Ferrand & R. Bloom (Eds.), *Introduction to organic and neurogenic disorders of communication* (pp. 110–138). Needham Heights, MA: Allyn & Bacon.

Coelho, C., DeRuyter, F., & Stein, M. (1996). Treatment efficacy: Cognitive-communicative disorders resulting from traumatic brain injury in adults. *Journal of Speech and Hearing Research, 39,* S5–S17.

Collins, M. (1983). Global aphasia: Knowledge in search of understanding. *Communication Disorders, 8,* 125–137.

Collins, M. (1991). *Diagnosis and treatment of global aphasia.* San Diego, CA: Singular.

Countryman, S., Hicks, J., Ramig, L., & Smith, M. (1997). Supraglottal hyperadduction in an individual with Parkinson disease: A clinical treatment note. *American Journal of Speech-Language Pathology, 6,* 74–84.

Crary, M., Haak, N., & Malinsky, A. (1989). Preliminary psychometric evaluation of an acute aphasia screening protocol. *Aphasiology, 3,* 611–618.

Creech, R., Wertz, R., & Rosenbek, J. (1973). Oral sensation and perception in dysarthric adults. *Perceptual & Motor Skills, 37,* 167–172.

Critchley, M. (1970). *Aphasiology and other aspects of language.* London: Edward Arnold.

Cummings, J. (1990). Introduction. In J. Cummings (Ed.), *Subcortical dementia* (pp. 3–16). New York: Oxford University Press.

Cummings, J., & Benson, D. (1992). *Dementia: A clinical approach* (2nd ed.). Stoneham, MA: Butterworth-Heinemann.

Dabul, B. (1979). *Apraxia Battery for Adults.* Tigard, OR: CC Publications.

Dabul, B., & Bollier, B. (1976). Therapeutic approaches to apraxia. *Journal of Speech and Hearing Disorders, 41,* 268–276.

Dalla Barba, G. (1993). Different patterns of confabulation. *Cortex, 29,* 567–581.

Damasio, A. (1991). Signs of aphasia. In M. Sarno (Ed.), *Acquired aphasia* (pp. 27–43). New York: Academic Press.

Damasio, H. (1991). Neuroanatomical correlates of the aphasias. In M. Sarno (Ed.), *Acquired aphasia* (pp. 45–71). New York: Academic Press.

Damecour, C., & Caplan, D. (1991). The relationship of depression to symptomatology and lesion site in aphasic patients. *Cortex, 27,* 385–401.

Darby, J., Simmons, N., & Berger, P. (1984). Speech and voice parameters of depression: A pilot study. *Journal of Communication Disorders, 17,* 75–85.

Darkins, A., Fromkin, V., & Benson, D. (1988). A characterization of the prosodic loss in Parkinson's disease. *Brain & Language, 34,* 315–327.

Darley, F. (1964). *Diagnosis and appraisal of communicative disorders.* Englewood Cliffs, NJ: Prentice-Hall.

Darley, F. (1972). The efficacy of language rehabilitation in aphasia. *Journal of Speech and Hearing Disorders, 37,* 3–21.

Darley, F. (1982). *Aphasia.* Philadelphia: Saunders.

Darley, F., Aronson, A., & Brown, J. (1969a). Clusters of deviant speech dimensions in the dysarthrias. *Journal of Speech and Hearing Research, 12,* 462–496.

Darley, F., Aronson, A., & Brown, J. (1969b). Differential diagnostic patterns of dysarthria. *Journal of Speech and Hearing Research, 12,* 246–269.

Darley, F., Aronson, A., & Brown, J. (1975). *Motor speech disorders.* Philadelphia: Saunders.

Darley, F., Brown, J., & Goldstein, N. (1972). Dysarthria in multiple sclerosis. *Journal of Speech and Hearing Research, 15,* 229–245.

David, R., Enderby, P., & Bainton, D. (1982). Treatment of acquired aphasia: Speech therapists and volunteers compared. *Journal of Neurology, Neurosurgery, and Psychiatry, 45,* 957–961.

Davis, G. (1993). *A survey of adult aphasia and related language disorders.* Englewood Cliffs, NJ: Prentice-Hall.

Davis, G., & Wilcox, J. (1981). Incorporating parameters of natural conversation in aphasia treatment. In R. Chapey (Ed.), *Language intervention strategies in adult aphasia* (pp. 169–193). Baltimore: Williams & Wilkins.

Day, L., & Parnell, M. (1987). Ten year study of a Wilson's disease dysarthric. *Journal of Communication Disorders, 20,* 207–218.

Deal, J. (1974). Consistency and adaptation in apraxia of speech. *Journal of Communication Disorders, 7,* 135–140.

Deal, J., & Darley, F. (1972). The influence of linguistic and situational variables on phonemic accuracy in apraxia of speech. *Journal of Speech and Hearing Research, 15,* 639–653.

Deal, J., & Deal, L. (1978). Efficacy of aphasia rehabilitation; preliminary results. In R. Brookshire (Ed.), *Clinical aphasiology conference proceedings* (pp. 66–67). Minneapolis, MN: BRK Publishers.

Deal, J., & Florance, C. (1978). Modification of the eight-step continuum for treatment of apraxia of speech in adults. *Journal of Speech and Hearing Disorders, 43,* 89–95.

Dementia. (1995, November). *Mayo Clinic Health Letter, 11,* 13.

DePaul, R, & Brooks, R. (1993). Multiple orofacial indices in amyotrophic lateral sclerosis. *Journal of Speech and Hearing Research, 36,* 1158–1167.

DeRenzi, E., & Ferrari, C. (1978). The Reporters Test: A sensitive test to detect expressive disturbances in aphasics. *Cortex, 14,* 279–293.

DeRenzi, E., Piezcuro, A., & Vignolo, L. (1966). Oral apraxia and aphasia. *Cortex, 2,* 50–73.

DeRenzi, E., & Vignolo, L. (1962). The Token Test: a sensitive test to detect receptive disturbances in aphasics. *Brain, 85,* 665–678.

DeSanti, S. (1997). Differentiating the dementias. In C. Ferrand and R. Bloom (Eds.), *Introduction to organic and neurogenic disorders of communication* (pp. 84–109). Needham Heights, MA: Allyn & Bacon.

Deutsch, S. (1981). Oral form identification as a measure of cortical sensory dysfunction, in apraxia of speech and aphasia. *Journal of Communication Disorders, 14,* 65–73.

Deutsch, S. (1984). Prediction of site of lesion from speech apraxic error patterns. In J. Rosenbek, M. McNeil, & A. Aronson (Eds.), *Apraxia of speech: Physiology, acoustics, linguistics management* (pp. 113–134). San Diego, CA: College Hill Press.

Dick, M., Kean, M., & Sands, D. (1989). Memory for internally generated words in Alzheimer-type dementia: Breakdown in encoding and semantic memory. *Brain & Cognition, 9,* 88–108.

DiSimoni, F. (1989). *Comprehensive Apraxia Test* (CAT). Dalton, PA: Praxis House.

DiSimoni, F., & Darley, F. (1977). Effect on phoneme duration control through utterance-length conditions in an apractic patient. *Journal of Speech and Hearing Disorders, 42,* 257–264.

DiSimoni, F., Darley, F., & Aronson, A. (1977). Patterns of dysfunction in schizophrenic patients on an aphasia test battery. *Journal of Speech and Hearing Disorders, 42,* 498–513.

Dromey, C., Ramig, L., & Johnson, A. (1995). Phonatory and articulatory changes associated with increased vocal intensity in Parkinson disease: A case study. *Journal of Speech and Hearing Research, 38,* 751–764.

Drummond, S. (1984). *Characterization of irrelevant speech: A case study.* Unpublished manuscript, University of Arkansas for Medical Science, Little Rock, AR.

Drummond, S. (1986). Characterization of irrelevant speech. *Journal of Communication Disorders, 19,* 175–183.

Duffy, J. (1994). Schuell's stimulation approach to rehabilitation. In R. Chapey (Ed.), *Language intervention strategies in adult aphasia* (pp. 146–174). Baltimore: Williams & Wilkins.

Duffy, J. (1995). *Motor speech disorders: Substrates, differential diagnosis and management.* St. Louis, MO: Mosby Yearbook.

Duffy, J., & Peterson, R. (1992). Primary progressive aphasia. *Aphasiology, 6,* 1–16.

Dunlop, J., & Marquardt, T. (1977). Linguistic and articulatory aspects of single word production in apraxia of speech. *Cortex, 13,* 17–29.

Dworkin, J. (1991). *Motor speech disorders: A treatment guide.* St. Louis, MO: Mosby.

Dworkin, J., Abkarian, G., & Johns, D. (1988). Apraxia of speech: The effectiveness of a treatment regimen. *Journal of Speech and Hearing Disorders, 53,* 280–294.

Dworkin, J., and Aronson, A. (1986). Tongue strength and alternate motion rates in normal and dysarthric subjects. *Journal of Communication Disorders, 19,* 115–132.

Dworkin, J., Aronson, A., & Mulder, D. (1980). Tongue force in normals and in dysarthric patients with amyotrophic lateral sclerosis. *Journal of Speech and Hearing Research, 23,* 828–837.

Dworkin J., & Culatta, R. (1980). *Dworkin-Culatta Oral Mechanism Examination.* Vero Beach, FL: Speech Bin.

Ehrlich, J. (1988). Selective characteristics of narrative discourse in head-injured and normal adults. *Journal of Communication Disorders, 21,* 1–9.

Eisenson, J. (1954). *Examining for aphasia.* New York: Psychological Corp.

Elman, R., & Bernstein-Ellis, E. (1999). The efficacy of group communication treatment in adults with chronic aphasia. *Journal of Speech-Language-Hearing Research, 42,* 411–419.

Enderby, P. (1983). *Frenchay Dysarthria Assessment.* San Diego, CA: College Hill Press.

Eustache, F., Lambert, J., Cassier, C., Dary, M., Rossa, Y., Rioux, P., Viader, F., & Lechevalier, B. (1995). Disorders of auditory identification in dementia of the Alzheimer type. *Cortex, 31,* 119–127.

Filley, C., & Kelly, J. (1990). Neurobehavioral effects of focal subcortical lesions. In J. Cummings (Ed.), *Subcortical dementia* (pp. 59–70). New York: Oxford University Press.

Fitch-West, J., & Sands, E. (1987). *The Bedside Evaluation Screening Test (BEST)*. Frederick, MD: Aspen.

Foldi, N. (1987). Appreciation of pragmatic interpretation of indirect commands: A comparison of right and left hemisphere brain-damaged patients. *Brain & Language, 31,* 88–108.

Folstein, M., Folstein, S., & McHugh, P. (1975). Mini-mental state: A practical guide for grading the mental state of patients for the clinician. *Journal of Psychiatric Research, 12,* 189–198.

Forrest, K., & Weismer, G. (1995). Dynamic aspects of lower lip movement in Parkinsonian and neurologically normal geriatric speakers' production of stress. *Journal of Speech and Hearing Research, 38,* 260–272.

Fox, C., & Ramig, L. (1997). Vocal sound pressure level and self-perception of speech and voice in men and women with idiopathic Parkinson disease. *American Journal of Speech-Language Pathology, 6,* 85–94.

Freed, D., & Marshall, R. (1995). The effect of personalized cueing on long term naming of realistic visual stimuli. *American Journal of Speech-Language Pathology, 4,* 105–108.

Freed, D., Marshall, R., & Nippold, M. (1995). Comparison of personalized cueing on the facilitation of verbal labeling by aphasic subjects. *Journal of Speech and Hearing Research, 38,* 1081–1090.

Froeschels, E. (1952). Chiming method as therapy. *Archives of Otolaryngology, 56,* 427–434.

Froeschels, E., Kastein, S., & Weiss, D. (1955). A method of therapy for paralytic conditions of the mechanisms of phonation, respiration, and glutination. *Journal of Speech and Hearing Disorders, 20,* 365–370.

Fromm, D., & Holland, A. (1989). Functional communication in Alzheimer's disease. *Journal of Speech and Hearing Disorders, 54,* 535–540.

Fromm, D., Holland, A., Nebes, R., & Oakley, M. (1991). A longitudinal study of word reading ability in Alzheimer's disease: Evidence from the National Adult Reading Test. *Cortex, 27*, 367–376.

Fuchs, E. (1981). *Comprehension of explicit and implicit information in adult aphasia.* Unpublished doctoral dissertation, Columbia University, New York.

Gandour, J., Holasuit Petty, S., & Dardarananda, R. (1988). Perception and production of tone in aphasia. *Brain & Language, 35*, 201–240.

Garcia, J., & Cannito, M. (1996). Influence of verbal and non-verbal contexts on the sentence intelligibility of a speaker with dysarthria. *Journal of Speech and Hearing Research, 39*, 750–760.

Garcia, J., & Dagenais, P. (1998). Dysarthric sentence intelligibility: Contribution of iconic gestures and message predictiveness. *Journal of Speech-Language-Hearing Research, 41*, 1282–1293.

Gardner, H., Zurif, E., Berry, T., & Baker, E. (1976). Visual communication in aphasia. *Neuropsychologia, 14*, 275–292.

Gentil, M. (1990). Dysarthria in Friedreich disease. *Brain & Language, 3*(8), 438–448.

Gerber, S., & Gurland, G. (1989). Applied pragmatics in the assessment of aphasia. *Seminars in Speech and Language*, 263–281.

Geschwind, N. (1967). The varieties of naming errors. *Cortex, 3*, 97–112.

Gewirth, L., Shindler, A., & Hier, D. (1984). Altered patterns of word associations in dementia and aphasia. *Brain & Language, 21*, 307–317.

Goldfarb, R., & Halpern, H. (1981). Word associations of time-altered auditory and visual stimuli in aphasia. *Journal of Speech and Hearing Research, 24*, 233–246.

Goldfarb, R., & Halpern, H. (1989). Impairments of naming and word finding. In C. Code (Ed.), *The characteristics of aphasia* (pp. 33–52). New York: Taylor & Francis.

Golper, L., & Cherney, L. (1999). Back to basics: Assessment practices with neurogenic communication disorders. *Neurophysiology and neurogenic speech and language disorders, 9*(3). [Special Interest Division Newsletter; Rockville, MD: American Speech-Language-Hearing Association].

Golper, L., Nutt, J., Rau, M., & Coleman, R. (1983). Focal cranial dystonia. *Journal of Speech and Hearing Disorders, 48,* 128–134.

Goodglass, H., & Kaplan, E. (1983). *Boston Diagnostic Aphasia Examination.* Philadelphia: Lea & Febiger.

Gordon-Adams, E. (1985). *Group counseling experiences and the self-reported behaviors and perceptions of wives of adult aphasics.* Unpublished doctoral dissertation, Columbia University, New York.

Goulet, P., & Joanette, Y. (1994). Sentence completion task in right-brain damaged right-handers: Eisenson's study revisited. *Brain & Language, 46,* 257–277.

Granholm, E., & Butters, N. (1988). Associative encoding and retrieval in Alzheimer's and Huntington's disease. *Brain & Cognition, 7,* 335–347.

Groher, M. (1977). Language and memory disorders following closed head trauma. *Journal of Speech and Hearing Research, 20,* 212–223.

Gruen, A., Frankle, B., & Schwartz, R. (1990). Word fluency generation skills of head-injured patients in an acute trauma center. *Journal of Communication Disorders, 23,* 163–170.

Gutbrod, K., Cohen, R., Maier, T., & Maier, E. (1987). Memory for spatial and temporal order in aphasic and right hemisphere damaged patients. *Cortex, 23,* 463–474.

Hagen, C. (1984). Language disorders in head trauma. In A. Holland (Ed.), *Language disorders in adults: Recent advances* (pp. 245–281). San Diego, CA: College Hill Press.

Halliday, M., & Hasan, R. (1976). *Cohesion in English.* London: Longman.

Halpern, H. (1965a). Effect of stimulus variables on dysphasic verbal errors. *Perceptual and Motor Skills, 21,* 291–298.

Halpern, H. (1965b). Effect of stimulus variables on verbal perseveration of dysphasic subjects. *Perceptual and Motor Skills, 20,* 421–429.

Halpern, H. (1986). *Language and motor speech disorders in adults.* Austin, TX: PRO-ED.

Halpern, H., Darley, F., & Brown, J. (1973). Differential language and neurologic characteristics in cerebral involvement. *Journal of Speech and Hearing Disorders, 38,* 162–173.

Halpern, H., Hochberg, I., & Rees, N. (1967). Speech and hearing characteristics in familial dysautonomia. *Journal of Speech and Hearing Research, 10,* 361–366.

Halpern, H., Keith, R., & Darley, F. (1976). Phonemic behavior of aphasic subjects without dysarthria or apraxia of speech. *Cortex, 12,* 365–372.

Halpern, H., & McCartin-Clark, M. (1984). Differential language characteristics in adult aphasic and schizophrenic subjects. *Journal of Communication Disorders, 17,* 289–307.

Hammarberg, B., Fritzell, B., & Schiratzki, H. (1984). Teflon injection in 16 patients with paralytic dysphonia: Perceptual and acoustic evaluation. *Journal of Speech and Hearing Disorders, 49,* 78–82.

Hammen, V., Yorkston, K., & Minifie, F. (1994). Effects of temporal alterations on speech intelligibility on Parkinsonian dysarthria. *Journal of Speech and Hearing Research, 37,* 244–253.

Hardison, D., Marquardt, T., & Peterson, H. (1977). Effects of selected linguistic variables on apraxia of speech. *Journal of Speech and Hearing Research, 20,* 334–343.

Hardy, J., Netsell, R., Schweiger, J., & Morris, H. (1969). Management of velopharyngeal dysfunction in cerebral palsy. *Journal of Speech and Hearing Disorders, 34,* 123–136.

Hartelius, L., Buder, E., & Strand, E. (1997). Long-term phonatory instability in individuals with multiple sclerosis. *Journal of Speech, Language, and Hearing Research, 40,* 1056–1072.

Hartley, L. (1994). Linguistic deficits after traumatic brain injury. *Neurophysiology and neurogenic speech and language disorders, 4*(1). [Special Interest Division Newsletter; Rockville, MD: American Speech-Language-Hearing Association].

Hartman, J., & Landau, W. (1987). Comparison of formal language therapy with supportive counseling for aphasia due to vascular accident. *Archives of Neurology, 44,* 646–649.

Haynes, W., Pindzola, R., & Emerick, L. (1992). *Diagnosis and evaluation in speech pathology.* Englewood Cliffs, NJ: Prentice-Hall.

Hearst Business Communications, Inc., RAI Division (n.d.). *Improving your ability to recall information.* New York: Author.

Hecaen, H. (1972). *Introduction a la neuropsychologie* [*Introduction to neuropsychology*]. Paris: Larousse.

Hegde, M. (1998). *A coursebook on aphasia.* San Diego, CA: Singular.

Heilman, K. (1994). Unpublished memo. Academy of Neurologic Communication Disorders and Sciences (ANCDS), Washington, DC.

Helm, N., & Barresi, B. (1980). Voluntary control of involuntary utterances: A treatment approach for severe aphasia. In R. Brookshire (Ed.), *Clinical aphasiology conference proceedings* (pp. 308–315 Minneapolis, MN: BRK Publishers.

Helm-Estabrooks, N. (1981). *Helm elicited language program for syntax stimulation* (HELPSS). Chicago: Riverside.

Helm-Estabrooks, N., Fitzpatric, P., & Barresi, B. (1982). Visual action therapy for global aphasia. *Journal of Speech and Hearing Disorders, 47,* 385–389.

Helm-Estabrooks, N., & Hotz, G. (1990). *The Brief Test of Head Injury* (BTHI). Austin, TX: PRO-ED.

Helm-Estabrooks, N., Ramsberger, G., Morgan, A., & Nicholas, M. (1989). *Boston Assessment of Severe Aphasia* (BASA). Chicago: Riverside.

Helmick, J., Watamori, T., & Palmer, J. (1976). Spouses' understanding of the communication disabilities of aphasic patients. *Journal of Speech and Hearing Disorders, 41,* 238–243.

Hier, D., Hagenlocker, K., & Shindler, A. (1985). Language disintegration in dementia: Effects of etiology and severity. *Brain & Language, 25,* 117–133.

Hirose, H. (1986). Pathophysiology of motor speech disorders (dysarthria). *Folia Phoniatrica, 38,* 61–68.

Hirose, H., Kiritani, S., & Sawashima, M. (1982). Patterns of dysarthric movement in patients with amyotrophic lateral sclerosis and pseudo-bulbar palsy. *Folia Phoniatrica, 34,* 106–112.

Hirose, H., Kiritani, S., Ushijima, T., & Sawashima, M. (1978). Analysis of abnormal articulatory dynamics in two dysarthric patients. *Journal of Speech and Hearing Disorders, 43,* 96–105.

Hixon, T., Putnam, A., & Sharp, J. (1983). Speech production with flaccid paralysis of the rib cage, diaphragm, and abdomen. *Journal of Speech and Hearing Disorders, 48,* 315–327.

Hoit, J., Banzett, R., Brown, R., & Loring, S. (1990). Speech breathing in individuals with cervical spinal cord injury. *Journal of Speech and Hearing Research, 33,* 798–807.

Hoit, J., & Shea, S. (1996). Speech production and speech with a phrenic nerve pacer. *American Journal of Speech-Language Pathology, 5,* 53–60.

Holland, A. (1970). Case studies in aphasia rehabilitation using programmed instructions. *Journal of Speech and Hearing Disorders, 35,* 377–390.

Holland, A. (1980). *Communication abilities in daily living.* Baltimore: University Park Press.

Holland, A., Fromm, D., DeRuyter, F., & Stein, M. (1996). Treatment efficacy: Aphasia. *Journal of Speech and Hearing Research, 39,* S27–S36.

Holland, A., McBurney, D., Moossy, J., & Reinmuth, O. (1985). The dissolution of language in Pick's disease with neurofibrillary tangles: A case study. *Brain & Language, 24,* 36–58.

Hoodin, R., & Gilbert, H. (1989). Nasal airflow in Parkinsonian speakers. *Journal of Communication Disorders, 22,* 169–180.

Horner, J., Dawson, D., Heyman, A., & Fish, A. (1992). The usefulness of the Western Aphasia Battery for differential diagnosis of Alzheimer dementia and focal stroke syndromes: Preliminary evidence. *Brain & Language, 42,* 77–88.

Horner, J., Heipman, A., Aker, C., Kanter, J., & Royall, J. (1982, October). *Misnamings of Alzheimer's dementia compared to misnaming associated with left and right hemisphere stroke.* Paper presented at the meeting of the Academy of Aphasia, New Paltz, NY.

Hough, M. (1990). Narrative comprehension in adults with right and left hemisphere brain damage: Theme organization. *Brain & Language, 38,* 253–277.

Hough, M. (1993). Treatment of Wernicke's aphasia with jargon: A case study. *Journal of Communication Disorders, 26,* 101–111.

Hough, M., & Klich, R. (1998). Lip EMG activity during vowel production in apraxia of speech: Phrase context and word length effects. *Journal of Speech-Language-Hearing Research, 41,* 786–801.

Hough, M., Pierce, R., & Cannito, M. (1989). Contextual influences in aphasia: Effects of predictive and nonpredictive narratives. *Brain & Language, 36,* 325–334.

Huber, S., & Shuttleworth, E. (1990). Neuropsychological assessment of subcortical dementia. In J. Cummings (Ed.), *Subcortical dementia* (pp. 71–86). New York: Oxford University Press.

Huff, F., Corkin, S., & Growdon, J. (1986). Semantic impairment and anomia in Alzheimer's disease. *Brain & Language, 28,* 235–249.

Huff, F., Mack, L., Mahlmann, J., & Greenberg, S. (1988). A comparison of lexical-semantic impairments in left hemisphere stroke and Alzheimer's disease. *Brain & Language, 34,* 262–278.

Hugdahl, K., Wester, K., & Asbjornsen, A. (1991). Auditory neglect after right frontal lobe and right pulvinar thalamic lesions. *Brain & Language, 41,* 465–473.

Hunt, K. (1965). *Grammatical structures written at three grade levels* (Research report #3). Champaign, IL: National Council of Teachers of English.

Jacobs, H. (1992). Behavior disorders and traumatic brain injury. *Neurophysiology and neurogenic speech and language disorders, 2*(1). [Special Interest Division Newsletter; Rockville, MD: American Speech-Language-Hearing Association].

Jennett, B., & Teasdale, G. (1981). *Management of head injuries.* Philadelphia: F. A. Davis.

Johns, D., & Darley, F. (1970). Phonemic variability in apraxia of speech. *Journal of Speech and Hearing Research, 13,* 556–583.

Johnson, K., & Bourgeois, M. (1998). Language intervention for patients with dementia attending a respite program. *Neurophysiology and neurogenic speech and language disorders, 8*(4). [Special Interest Division Newsletter; Rockville, MD: American Speech-Language-Hearing Association].

Kahn, H., Stannard, T., & Skinner, J. (1998). The use of words versus nonwords in the treatment of apraxia of speech: A case study. *Neurophysiology and neurogenic speech and language disorders, 8*(3). [Special Interest Division Newsletter; Rockville, MD: American Speech-Language-Hearing Association].

Kangas, K., & Lloyd, L. (1998). Augmentative and alternative communication. In G. Shames, E. Wiig, & W. Secord (Eds.), *Human communication disorders: An introduction* (pp. 510–551). Needham Heights, MA: Allyn & Bacon.

Kaplan, E., Goodglass, H., & Weintraub, S. (1983). *The Boston Naming Test.* Philadelphia: Lea-Febiger.

Kaplan, J., Brownell, H., Jacobs, J., & Gardner, H. (1990). The effects of right hemisphere damage on the pragmatic interpretation of conversational remarks. *Brain & Language, 38,* 315–333.

Katz, R., & Wertz, R. (1997). The efficacy of computer-provided reading treatment for chronic aphasic adults. *Journal of Speech-Language-Hearing Research, 40,* 493–507.

Kearns, K. (1985). Response elaboration training for patient-initiated utterances. In R. Brookshire (Ed.), *Clinical aphasiology conference proceedings* (pp. 196–204). Minneapolis, MN: BRK.

Kearns, K. (1994). Group therapy for aphasia: Theoretical and practical considerations. In R. Chapey (Ed.), *Language intervention strategies in adult aphasia* (pp. 304–321). Baltimore: Williams & Wilkins.

Keenan, J., & Brassell, E. (1975). *Aphasia Language Performance Scales.* Murfreesboro, TN: Pinnacle Press.

Keith, R., & Aronson, A. (1975). Singing as therapy for apraxia of speech and aphasia: Report of a case. *Brain & Language, 2,* 483.

Keith, R., & Thomas, J. (1989). *Speech practice manual for dysarthria, apraxia, and other disorders of articulation.* Philadelphia: Decker.

Keller, E. (1984). Simplification and gesture reduction in phonological disorders of apraxia and aphasia. In J. Rosenbek, M. McNeil, & A. Aronson (Eds.), *Apraxia of speech: Physiology, acoustics, linguistics, management* (pp. 221–256). San Diego, CA: College Hill Press.

Kempler, D., Curtiss, S., & Jackson, C. (1987). Syntactic preservation in Alzheimer's disease. *Journal of Speech and Hearing Research, 30,* 343–350.

Kent, J., Kent, R., Rosenbek, J., Weismer, G., Martin, R., Sufit, R., & Brooks, B. (1992). Quantitative description of the dysarthria in women with amyotrophic lateral sclerosis. *Journal of Speech and Hearing Research, 35,* 723–733.

Kent, R. (1997). *The speech sciences.* San Diego, CA: Singular.

Kent, R., Kent, J., Weismer, G., Sufit, R., Rosenbek, J., Martin, R., & Brooks, B. (1990). Impairment of speech intelligibility in men with amyotrophic lateral sclerosis. *Journal of Speech and Hearing Disorders, 55,* 721–728.

Kent, R., & Netsell, R. (1978). Articulatory abnormalities in athetoid cerebral palsy. *Journal of Speech and Hearing Disorders, 43,* 353–373.

Kent, R., & Rosenbek, J. (1983). Acoustic patterns of apraxia of speech. *Journal of Speech and Hearing Research, 26,* 231–249.

Kent, R., Sufit, R., Rosenbek, J., Kent, J., Weismer, G., Martin, R., & Brooks, B. (1991). Speech deterioration in amyotrophic lateral sclerosis: Case study. *Journal of Speech and Hearing Research, 34,* 1269–1275.

Kent, R., Weismer, G., Kent, J., & Rosenbek, J. (1989). Toward phonetic intelligibility testing in dysarthria. *Journal of Speech and Hearing Disorders, 54,* 482–499.

Kertesz, A. (1982). *The Western Aphasia Battery.* New York: Gruen & Stratton.

Kertesz, A. (1984). Subcortical lesions and verbal apraxia. In J. Rosenbek, M. McNeil, & A. Aronson (Eds.), *Apraxia of speech: Physiology, acoustics, linguistics, management* (pp. 73–90). San Diego, CA: College Hill Press.

Kertesz, A., Lau, W., & Polk, M. (1993). The structural determinants of recovery in Wernicke's aphasia. *Brain & Language, 44,* 153–164.

Kilpatrick, K., & Jones, C. (1977). *Therapy guide for language and speech disorders.* Akron, OH: Visiting Nurse Service.

Kimelman, M. (1991). The role of target word stress in auditory comprehension by aphasic listeners. *Journal of Speech and Hearing Research, 34,* 334–339.

King, J., & Hux, K. (1996). Attention allocation in adults with and without aphasia: Performance on linguistic and nonlinguistic tasks. *American Journal of Medical Speech-Language Pathology, 4,* 245–256.

Klich, R., Ireland, J., & Weidner, W. (1979). Articulatory and chronological aspects of consonant substitution in apraxia of speech. *Cortex, 15,* 451–470.

Kontiola, P., Laaksonen, R., Sulkava, R., & Erkin-Juntti, T. (1990). Pattern of language impairment is different in Alzheimer's disease and multi-infarct dementia. *Brain & Language, 38,* 364–383.

LaBlance, G., & Rutherford, D. (1991). Respiratory dynamics and speech intelligibility in speakers with generalized dystonia. *Journal of Communication Disorders, 24,* 141–156.

Langmore, S., & Lehman, M. (1994). Physiologic deficits in the orofacial system underlying dysarthria in amyotrophic lateral sclerosis. *Journal of Speech and Hearing Research, 37,* 28–37.

LaPointe, L. (1977). Base-10 programmed stimulation: Task specification scoring and plotting performance in aphasia therapy. *Journal of Speech and Hearing Disorders, 42,* 90–105.

LaPointe, L., & Horner, J. (1976). Repeated trials of words by patients with neurogenic phonological selection-sequencing impairment (apraxia of speech). In R. Brookshire (Ed.), *Clinical aphasiology conference proceedings* (pp. 261–277). Minneapolis, MN: BRK Publishers.

LaPointe, L., & Horner, J. (1980). *Reading Comprehension Battery for Aphasia.* Tigard, OR: C.C. Publications.

LaPointe, L., & Johns, D. (1975). Some phonetic characteristics in apraxia of speech. *Journal of Communication Disorders, 8,* 259–269.

LaPointe, L., & Katz, R. (1998). Neurogenic disorders of speech. In G. Shames, E. Wiig, & W. Secord (Eds.), *Human communication disor-*

ders: An introduction (pp. 434–471). Needham Heights, MA: Allyn & Bacon.

LaPointe, L., & Wertz, R. (1974). Oral-movement abilities and articulatory characteristics of brain-injured adults. *Perceptual and Motor Skills, 39,* 39–46.

Lass, N., Ruscello, D., Harkins, K., & Blankenship, B. (1993). A comparative study of adolescents' perceptions of normal-speaking and dysarthric children. *Journal of Communication Disorders, 26,* 3–12.

Lass, N., Ruscello, D., & Lakawicz, J. (1988). Listeners' perceptions of non-speech characteristics of normal and dysarthric children. *Journal of Communication Disorders, 21,* 385–391.

LeDorze, G., Ouellet, L., & Ryalls, J. (1994). Intonation and speech rate in dysarthric speech. *Journal of Communication Disorders, 27,* 1–18.

Levin, H., O'Donnell, V., & Grossman, R. (1979). The Galveston Orientation and Amnesia Test: A practice scale to assess cognition after head injury. *Journal of Nervous and Mental Disease, 167,* 675–684.

Lezak, M. (1982). The problem of assessing executive functions. *International Journal of Psychology, 17,* 281–297.

Li, E., & Williams, S. (1990). Repetition deficits in three aphasic syndromes. *Journal of Communication Disorders, 23,* 77–88.

Liles, B., Coelho, C., Duffy, R., & Zalagens, M. (1989). Effects of elicitation procedures on the narratives of normal and closed head injured adults. *Journal of Speech and Hearing Disorders, 54,* 356–366.

Lincoln, N., Mulley, G., Jones, A., McGurik, E., Lendrem, W., & Mitchell, J. (1984, June). Effectiveness of speech therapy for aphasic stroke patients: A randomized controlled trial. *The Lancet, 1,* 1197–1200.

Linebaugh, C. (1979). The dysarthrias of Shy-Drager syndrome. *Journal of Speech and Hearing Disorders, 44,* 55–60.

Linebaugh, C., & Wolfe, V. (1984). Relationships between articulation rate, intelligibility, and naturalness in spastic and ataxic speakers. In M. McNeil, J. Rosenbek, & A. Aronson (Eds.), *The dysarthrias: Physiology, acoustics, perception, management* (pp. 195–205). San Diego, CA: College Hill Press.

Logemann, J., & Fisher, H. (1981). Vocal tract control in Parkinson's disease: Phonetic feature analysis of misarticulations. *Journal of Speech and Hearing Disorders, 46,* 348–352.

Logemann, J., Fisher, H., Boshes, B., & Blonsky, E. (1978). Frequency and cooccurrence of vocal tract dysfunctions in the speech of a large sample of Parkinson patients. *Journal of Speech and Hearing Disorders, 43,* 47–57.

Lomas, J., Picard, I., Bester, S., Elbard, H., Finlayson, A., & Zoghaib, C. (1989). The Communicative Effectiveness Index: Development and psychometric evaluation of a functional communication measure for adult aphasia. *Journal of Speech and Hearing Disorders, 54,* 113–124.

Love, R., Hagerman, E., & Taimi, E. (1980). Speech performance, dysphagia and oral reflexes in cerebral palsy. *Journal of Speech and Hearing Disorders, 45,* 59–75.

Love, R., & Webb, W. (1996). *Neurology for the speech-language pathologist.* Woburn, MA: Butterworth-Heinemann.

Lowell, S., Beeson, P., & Holland, A. (1995). The efficacy of a semantic cueing procedure on naming performance of adults with aphasia. *American Journal of Speech-Language Pathology, 4*(4), 109–114.

Ludlow, C., Connor, N., & Bassich, C. (1987). Speech timing in Parkinson's and Huntington's disease. *Brain & Language, 32,* 195–214.

Lyon, J. (1992). Communication use and participation in life for adults with aphasia in natural settings: The scope of the problem. *American Journal of Speech-Language Pathology, 1*(3), 7–14.

Marcie, P., Roudier, M., Goldblum, M., & Boller, F. (1993). Principal component analysis of language performances in Alzheimer's disease. *Journal of Communication Disorders, 26,* 53–63.

Marquardt, T., Reinhart, J., & Peterson, H. (1979). Markedness analysis of phonemic substitution errors in apraxia of speech. *Journal of Communication Disorders, 12,* 481–494.

Marquardt, T., & Sussman, H. (1984). The elusive lesion—apraxia of speech link in Broca's aphasia. In J. Rosenbek, M. McNeil, & A. Aronson (Eds.), *Apraxia of speech: Physiology, acoustics, linguistics, management* (pp. 91–112). San Diego, CA: College Hill Press.

Marshall, R. (1993). Problem-focused group treatment for clients with mild aphasia. *American Journal of Speech-Language Pathology, 2*(2), 31–37.

Marshall, R., & Tompkins, C. (1981). Identifying behavior associated with verbal self-corrections of aphasic clients. *Journal of Speech and Hearing Disorders, 46,* 168–173.

Marshall, R., Wertz, R., Weiss, D., Aten, J., Brookshire, R., Garcia-Bunuel, L., Holland, A., Kurtzke, J., LaPointe, L., Milianti, F., Brannigan, R., Greenbaum, H., Vogel, D., Carter, J., Barnes, N., & Goodman, P. (1989). Home treatment for aphasic patients by trained non professionals. *Journal of Speech and Hearing Disorders, 54,* 462–470.

Martin, A., & Fedio, P. (1983). Word production and comprehension in Alzheimer's disease: The breakdown of semantic knowledge. *Brain & Language, 19,* 124–141.

Mateer, C. (1996). Managing impairments in attention following traumatic brain injury. *Neurophysiology and neurogenic speech and language disorders, 6*(3) [Special Interest Division Newsletter; Rockville, MD: American Speech-Language-Hearing Association].

Mathews, P., Obler, L., & Albert, M. (1994). Wernicke and Alzheimer on the language disturbances of dementia and aphasia. *Brain & Language, 46,* 439–462.

Mattis, S. (1976). Mental status examination for organic mental syndrome in the elderly patient. In R. Black & B. Karasu (Eds.), *Geriatric psychiatry* (pp. 77–121). New York: Gruen & Stratton.

McDonald, S., & Wales, R. (1986). An investigation of the ability to process inferences in language following right hemisphere brain damage. *Brain & Language, 29,* 68–80.

McKhann, G., Drachman, D., Folstein, M., Katzman, R., Price, D., & Stadlan, E. (1984). Clinical diagnosis of Alzheimer's disease: Report of the NINCDS-ADRDA work group under the auspices of the Dept. of Health and Human Services task force on Alzheimer's disease. *Neurology, 34,* 939–944.

McNamara, P., Obler, L., Au, R., Durso, R., & Albert, M. (1992). Speech monitoring skills in Alzheimer's disease, Parkinson's disease, and normal aging. *Brain & Language, 42,* 38–51.

McNamara, R. (1983). A conceptual holistic approach to dysarthria treatment. In W. Berry (Ed.), *Clinical dysarthria* (pp. 191–201). San Diego, CA: College Hill Press.

McNeil, M., Liss, J., Tseng, C., & Kent, R. (1990). Effects of speech rate on the absolute and relative timing of apraxic and conduction aphasic sentence production. *Brain & Language, 38,* 135–158.

McNeil, M., & Prescott, T. (1978). *Revised Token Test.* Baltimore: University Park Press.

McNeil, M., Small, S., Masterson, R., & Fossett, T. (1995). Behavioral and pharmacological treatment of lexical-semantic deficits in a single patient with primary progressive aphasia. *American Journal of Speech-Language Pathology, 4,* 76–87.

McNeil, M., Weismer, G., Adams, S., & Mulligan, M. (1990). Oral structure nonspeech motor control in normal, dysarthric, aphasic, and apraxic speakers: Isometric force and static position control. *Journal of Speech and Hearing Research, 33,* 255–268.

Meikle, M., Wechsler, E., Tupper, A., Benenson, M., Butler, J., Mulhall, D., & Stern, G. (1979). Comparative trial of volunteer and professional treatments of dysphasia after stroke. *British Medical Journal, 2,* 87–89.

Mentis, M., Briggs-Whitaker, J., & Gramigna, G. (1995). Discourse topic management in senile dementia of the Alzheimer's type. *Journal of Speech and Hearing Research, 38,* 1054–1066.

Mesulam, M. (1990). Large scale neurocognitive networks and distributed processing for attention, language and memory. *Annals of Neurology, 28,* 597–613.

Mills, R., & Drummond, S. (1980, November). *Analysis of impaired naming in language of confusion.* Paper presented at the meeting of the American Speech-Language-Hearing Association, Detroit, MI.

Mlcoch, A., & Metter, J. (1994). Medical aspects of stroke rehabilitation. In R. Chapey (Ed.), *Language intervention strategies in adult aphasia* (pp. 27–46). Baltimore: Williams & Wilkins.

Morris, R. (1987). Articulatory rehearsal in Alzheimer type dementia. *Brain & Language, 30,* 351–362.

Mosby medical encyclopedia. (1992). New York: Mosby.

Mosby medical, nursing, and allied health dictionary. (1994). St. Louis, MO: Mosby.

Mulligan, M., Carpenter, J., Riddel, J., Delaney, M., Badger, G., Krusinski, P., & Tandan, R. (1994). Intelligibility and the acoustic characteristics of speech in amyotrophic lateral sclerosis (ALS). *Journal of Speech and Hearing Research, 37,* 496–503.

Murdoch, B. (1990). *Acquired speech and language disorders.* London: Chapman and Hall.

Murdoch, B., Chenery, H., Stokes, P., & Hardcastle, W. (1991). Respiratory kinematics in speakers with cerebellar disease. *Journal of Speech and Hearing Research, 34,* 768–780.

Murdoch, B., Chenery, H., Wilks, V., & Boyle, R. (1987). Language disorders in dementia of the Alzheimer type. *Brain & Language, 31,* 122–137.

Murray, L., Holland, A., & Beeson, P. (1997). Auditory processing in individuals with mild aphasia: A study of resource allocation. *Journal of Speech-Language-Hearing Research, 40,* 792–808.

Murray, L., Holland, A., & Beeson, P. (1998). Spoken language of individuals with mild fluent aphasia under focused and divided-attention conditions. *Journal of Speech-Language-Hearing Research, 41,* 213–227.

Murry, T. (1978). Speaking fundamental frequency characteristics associated with voice pathologies. *Journal of Speech and Hearing Disorders, 43,* 374–379.

Murry, T. (1984). Treatment for ataxic dysarthria. In W. Perkins (Ed.), *Dysarthria and apraxia* (pp. 75–89). New York: Thieme-Stratton.

Myers, P. (1986). Right hemisphere communication impairment. In R. Chapey (Ed.), *Language intervention strategies in adult aphasia* (pp. 444–461). Baltimore: Williams & Wilkins.

Myers, P. (1994). Communication disorders associated with right-hemisphere brain damage. In R. Chapey (Ed.), *Language intervention strategies in adult aphasia* (pp. 513–532). Baltimore: Williams & Wilkins.

Myers, P., & Brookshire, R. (1996). Effect of visual and inferential variables on scene descriptions by right-hemisphere-damaged and non-brain-damaged adults. *Journal of Speech and Hearing Research, 39,* 870–880.

Natsopoulos, D., Katsarov, Z., Bostantzopoulou, S., Grovious, G., Mentenopoulos, G., & Logothetis, J. (1991). Strategies in comprehension of relative clauses by Parkinsonian patients. *Cortex, 27,* 255–268.

Nebes, R., & Boller, F. (1987). The use of language structure by demented patients in a visual search task. *Cortex, 28,* 87–98.

Neils, J., Roeltgen, D., & Constantinidou, F. (1995). Decline in homophone spelling associated with loss of semantic influence on spelling in Alzheimer's disease. *Brain & Language, 49,* 27–49.

Nemec, R., & Cohen, K. (1984). EMG biofeedback in the modification of hypertonia in spastic dysarthria: Case report. *Archives of Physical Medicine and Rehabilitation, 65,* 103–104.

Netsell, R. (1984). A neurobiologic view of the dysarthrias. In M. McNeil, J. Rosenbek, & A. Aronson (Eds.), *The dysarthrias: Physiology, acoustics, perception, management* (pp. 1–36). San Diego, CA: College Hill Press.

Netsell, R. (1994). Instrumentation and special proceedings for individuals with dysarthria. *American Journal of Speech-Language Pathology, 3,* 9–11.

Netsell, R. (1995). Speech rehabilitation for individuals with unintelligible speech and dysarthria: The respiratory and velopharyngeal systems. *Neurophysiology and neurogenic speech and language disorders 2*(4) [Special Interest Division Newsletter; Rockville, MD: American Speech-Language-Hearing Association].

Netsell, R., & Lefkowitz, D. (1992). Speech production following traumatic brain injury: Clinical and research implications. *Neurophysiology and neurogenic speech and language disorders, 2*(4). [Special Interest Division Newsletter; Rockville, MD: American Speech-Language-Hearing Association].

Nicholas, L., & Brookshire, R. (1993). A system for quantifying the informativeness and efficiency of the connected speech of adults with aphasia. *Journal of Speech and Hearing Research, 36,* 338–350.

Nicholas, L., & Brookshire, R. (1995a). Comprehension of spoken narrative discourse by adults with aphasia, right-hemisphere brain damage, or traumatic brain injury. *American Journal of Speech-Language Pathology, 4,* 69–81.

Nicholas, L., & Brookshire, R. (1995b). Presence, completeness, and accuracy of main concepts in the connected speech of non-brain damaged adults and adults with aphasia. *Journal of Speech and Hearing Research, 38,* 145–156.

Nicholas, M., Obler, L., Albert, M., & Helm-Estabrooks, N. (1985). Empty speech in Alzheimer's disease and fluent aphasia. *Journal of Speech and Hearing Research, 28,* 405–410.

Obler, L., & Albert, M. (1981). Language in the elderly aphasic and in the dementing patient. In M. Sarno (Ed.), *Acquired aphasia* (pp. 385–398). New York: Academic Press.

Obler, L., Albert, M., Estabrooks, N., & Nicholas, M. (1982, October). *Noninformative speech in Alzheimer's dementia and in Wernicke's aphasia.* Paper presented at the meeting of the Academy of Aphasia, New Paltz, NY.

Ochipa, C., Maher, L., & Raymer, H. (1998). One approach to the treatment of anomia. *Neurophysiology and neurogenic speech and language disorders, 8*(3) [Special Interest Division Newsletter; Rockville, MD: American Speech-Language-Hearing Association].

Odell, K., McNeil, M., Rosenbek, J., & Hunter, L. (1990). Perceptual characteristics of consonant production by apraxic speakers. *Journal of Speech and Hearing Disorders, 55,* 345–359.

Odell, K., McNeil, M., Rosenbek, J., & Hunter, L. (1991). Perceptual characteristics of vowel and prosody production in apraxic, aphasic, and dysarthric speakers. *Journal of Speech and Hearing Research, 34,* 67–80.

O'Dwyer, N., Neilson, P., Guitar, B., Quinn, P., & Andrews, G. (1983). Control of upper airway structures during nonspeech tasks in normal and cerebral palsied subjects: EMG findings. *Journal of Speech and Hearing Research, 26,* 162–170.

Oelschlaeger, M. (1999). Participation of a conversation-partner in the word searches of a person with aphasia. *American Journal of Speech-Language Pathology, 8,* 62–71.

Orange, J., & Colton-Hudson, A. (1998). A case study of spousal communication education and training program for Alzheimer's disease. *Neurophysiology and neurogenic speech and language disorders, 8*(4) [Special Interest Division Newsletter; Rockville, MD: American Speech-Language-Hearing Association].

Orange, J., Lubinski, R., & Higginbotham, D. (1996). Conversational repair by individuals with dementia of the Alzheimer's type. *Journal of Speech and Hearing Research, 39,* 881–895.

Owens, R., & House, L. (1984). Decision-making processes in augmentative communication. *Journal of Speech and Hearing Disorders, 49,* 18–25.

Paradis, M. (1987). *The assessment of bilingual aphasia.* Hillsdale, NJ: Lawrence Erlbaum.

Peach, R. (1992). Factors underlying neuropsychological test performance in chronic severe traumatic brain injury. *Journal of Speech and Hearing Research, 35,* 810–818.

Peach, R., & Rubin, S. (1994). Treatment of global aphasia. In R. Chapey (Ed.), *Language intervention strategies in adult aphasia* (pp. 429–445). Baltimore: Williams & Wilkins.

Peterson, H., & Marquardt, T. (1994). *Appraisal and diagnosis of speech and language disorders.* Englewood Cliffs, NJ: Prentice-Hall.

Pimental, P., & Kingsbury, N. (1989). *Mini Inventory of Right Brain Injury.* Austin, TX: Pro-Ed.

Poeck, K., Huber, W., & Willmes, K. (1989). Outcome of intensive language treatment in aphasia. *Journal of Speech and Hearing Disorders, 54,* 471–479.

Porch, B. (1981). *Porch Index of Communicative Ability.* Palo Alto, CA: Consulting Psychologists Press.

Portnoy, R. (1979). Hyperkinetic dysarthria as an early indicator of impending tardive dyskinesia. *Journal of Speech and Hearing Disorders, 44,* 214–219.

Portnoy, R., & Aronson, A. (1982). Diadochokinetic syllable rate and regularity in normal and in spastic and ataxic dysarthric subjects. *Journal of Speech and Hearing Disorders, 47,* 324–328.

Prutting, C., & Kirchner, D. (1987). A clinical appraisal of the pragmatic aspects of language. *Journal of Speech and Hearing Disorders, 52,* 105–119.

Putnam, A., & Hixon, T. (1984). Respiratory kinematics in speakers with motor neuron disease. In M. McNeil, J. Rosenbek, & A. Aronson (Eds.), *The dysarthrias: Physiology, acoustics perception, management* (pp. 36–67). San Diego, CA: College Hill Press.

Rabins, P., Mace, N., & Lucas, M. (1982). The impact of dementia on the family. *Journal of the American Medical Association, 248,* 333–336.

Ramig, L. (1995). Speech treatment for individuals with Parkinson disease. *Neurophysiology and neurogenic speech and language disorders,* 5(4) [Special Interest Division Newsletter; Rockville, MD: American Speech-Language-Hearing Association].

Ramig, L., Countryman, S., Thompson, L., & Horii, Y. (1995). Comparison of two forms of intensive speech treatment for Parkinson disease. *Journal of Speech and Hearing Research, 38,* 1232–1251.

Ramig, L., & Dromey, C. (1996). Aerodynamic mechanisms underlying treatment related changes in vocal intensity in patients with Parkinson disease. *Journal of Speech and Hearing Research, 39,* 798–807.

Rehak, A., Kaplan, J., Weylman, S., Kelly, B., Brownell, H., & Gardner, H. (1992). Story processing in right-hemisphere brain-damaged patients. *Brain & Language, 42,* 320–336.

Reich, A., and Lerman, J. (1978). Teflon laryngoplasty: An acoustical and perceptual study. *Journal of Speech and Hearing Disorders, 43,* 496–505.

Reisberg, B., Ferris, S., DeLeon, M., & Crook, T. (1982). The Global Deterioration Scale (GDS): An instrument for the assessment of primary degenerative dementia (PDD). *American Journal of Psychiatry, 139,* 1136–1139.

Renout, K., Leeper, H., Bandur, D., & Hudson, A. (1995). Vocal fold diadochokinetic function of individuals with amyotrophic lateral sclerosis. *American Journal of Speech-Language Pathology, 4(1),* 73–80.

Reuterskiold, C. (1991). The effects of emotionality on auditory comprehension in aphasia. *Cortex, 27,* 595–604.

Riddel, J., McCauley, R., Mulligan, M., & Tandan, R. (1995). Intelligibility and phonetic contrast errors in highly intelligible speakers with amyotrophic lateral sclerosis. *Journal of Speech and Hearing Research, 38,* 304–314.

Ripich, D., & Terrell, B. (1988). Patterns of discourse, cohesion, and coherence in Alzheimer's disease. *Journal of Speech and Hearing Disorders, 53,* 8–15.

Robertson, I., Halligan, P., Bergego, C., Homberg, V., Pizzamiglio, L., Weber, E., & Wilson, B. (1994). Right neglect following right hemisphere damage? *Cortex, 30,* 199–213.

Robey, R. (1994). The efficacy of treatment for aphasic persons: A meta-analysis. *Brain & Language, 47,* 582–608.

Robey, R. (1998). A meta-analysis of clinical outcomes in the treatment of aphasia. *Journal of Speech, Language, and Hearing Research, 41,* 172–187.

Robin, D., Bean, C., & Folkins, J. (1989). Lip movement in apraxia of speech. *Journal of Speech and Hearing Research, 32,* 512–523.

Rochon, E., Waters, G., & Caplan, D. (1994). Sentence comprehension in patients with Alzheimer's disease. *Brain & Language, 46,* 329–349.

Roman, M., Brownell, H., Potter, M., Seibold, M., & Gardner, H. (1987). Script knowledge in right hemisphere damaged and normal elderly adults. *Brain & Language, 31,* 151–170.

Rosenbek, J. (1984). Treatment for apraxia of speech in adults. In W. Perkins (Ed.), *Dysarthria and apraxia* (pp. 49–56). New York: Thieme-Stratton.

Rosenbek, J. (1985). Treating apraxia of speech. In D. Johns (Ed.), *Clinical management of neurogenic communicative disorders* (pp. 267–312). Boston: Little, Brown.

Rosenbek, J., Hansen, R., Baughman, C., & Lemme, M. (1974). Treatment of developmental apraxia of speech: A case study. *Language Speech and Hearing Services in the Schools, 5,* 13–22.

Rosenbek, J., Kent, R., & LaPointe, L. (1984). Apraxia of speech: An overview and some perspectives. In J. Rosenbek, M. McNeil, & A. Aronson (Eds.), *Apraxia of speech: Physiology, acoustics, linguistics, management* (pp. 1–72). San Diego, CA: College Hill Press.

Rosenbek, J., & LaPointe, L. (1985). The dysarthrias: Description, diagnosis, and treatment. In D. Johns (Ed.), *Clinical management of neurogenic communicative disorders* (pp. 97–152). Boston: Little, Brown.

Rosenbek, J., LaPointe, L., & Wertz, R. (1989). *Aphasia: A clinical approach.* Boston: Little, Brown.

Rosenbek, J., Lemme, M., Ahern, M., Harris, E., & Wertz, R. (1973). A treatment for apraxia of speech in adults. *Journal of Speech and Hearing Disorders, 38,* 462–472.

Rosenbek, J., Wertz, R., & Darley, F. (1973). Oral sensation and perception in apraxia of speech. *Journal of Speech and Hearing Research, 16,* 22–36.

Ross-Swain, D. (1996). *Ross Information Processing Assessment* (2nd ed.). Austin, TX: Pro-Ed.

Rubow, R., Rosenbek, J., Collins, M., & Celesia, G. (1984). Reduction of hemifacial spasm and dysarthria following EMG biofeedback. *Journal of Speech and Hearing Disorders, 49,* 26–33.

Salvatore, A., & Thompson, C. (1986). Intervention for global aphasia. In R. Chapey (Ed.), *Language intervention strategies in adult aphasia* (pp. 402–418). Baltimore: Williams & Wilkins.

Samlan R., & Weismer, G. (1995). The relationship of selected perceptual measures of diadochokinesis to speech intelligibility in dysarthric speakers with amyotrophic lateral sclerosis. *American Journal of Speech-Language Pathology, 4,* 9–13.

Santo Pietro, M., & Goldfarb, R. (1985). Characteristic patterns of word association responses in institutionalized elderly with and without senile dementia. *Brain & Language, 26,* 230–243.

Santo Pietro, M., & Goldfarb, R. (1995). *Techniques for aphasia rehabilitation: Generating effective treatment* (TARGET). Vero Beach, FL: Speech Bin.

Sapir, S., & Aronson, A. (1990). The relationship between psychopathology and speech and language disorders in neurologic patients. *Journal of Speech and Hearing Disorders, 55,* 503–509.

Sarno, J. (1991). The psychological and social sequelae of aphasia. In M. Sarno (Ed.), *Acquired aphasia* (pp. 499–519). New York: Academic Press.

Sarno, M. (1969). *Functional communication profile.* New York: Institute of Rehabilitative Medicine.

Sarno, M. (1991). Recovery and rehabilitation in aphasia. In M. Sarno (Ed.), *Acquired aphasia* (pp. 521–582). New York: Academic Press.

Sarno, M., Buonaguro, A., & Levita, E. (1986). Characteristics of verbal impairment in CHI patients. *Archives of Physical Medicine and Rehabilitation, 67,* 400–405.

Sarno, M., Silverman, M., & Sands, E. (1970). Speech therapy and language recovery in severe aphasia. *Journal of Speech and Hearing Research, 13,* 607–623.

Schneiderman, E., Murasugi, K., & Saddy, J. (1992). Story arrangement ability in right-brain-damaged patients. *Brain & Language, 43,* 107–120.

Schuell, H. (1972). *The Minnesota Test for the Differential Diagnosis of Aphasia.* Minneapolis, MN: University of Minnesota Press.

Schuell, H., Jenkins, J., & Jimenez-Pabon, E. (1964). *Aphasia in adults: Diagnosis, prognosis, and treatment.* New York: Hoeber Medical Division, Harper.

Schulte, E., & Brandt, S. (1989). Auditory verbal comprehension impairment. In C. Code (Ed.), *The characteristics of aphasia* (pp. 53–74). Philadelphia: Taylor & Francis.

Schwartz, D., & Halpern, H. (1973). Effect of body-image stimuli on verbal errors of dysphasic subjects. *Perceptual and Motor Skills, 36,* 994.

Seddoh, S., Robin, D., Sim, H., Hageman, C., Moon, J., & Folkins, J. (1996). Speech timing in apraxia of speech versus conduction aphasia. *Journal of Speech and Hearing Research, 39,* 590–603.

Seikel, J., Wilcox, K., & Davis, J. (1990). Dysarthria of motor neuron disease: Clinician judgments of severity. *Journal of Communication Disorders, 23,* 417–431.

Shane, H., & Bashir, A. (1980). Election criterion for the adoption of an augmentative communication system, preliminary considerations. *Journal of Speech and Hearing Research, 45,* 408–414.

Shane, H., & Darley, F. (1978). The effect of auditory rhythmic stimulation on articulatory accuracy in apraxia of speech. *Cortex, 14,* 444–450.

Shane, H., & Sauer, M. (1986). *Augmentative and alternative communication.* Austin, TX: PRO-ED.

Shankweiler, D., & Harris, K. (1966). An experimental approach to the problem of articulation in aphasia. *Cortex, 2,* 277–292.

Shaughnessy, A., Netsell, R., & Farrage, J. (1983). Treatment of a four-year old with a palatal lift prosthesis. In W. Berry (Ed.), *Clinical dysarthria* (pp. 217–230). San Diego, CA: College Hill Press.

Sheard, C., Adams, R., & Davis, P. (1991). Reliability and agreement of ratings of ataxic dysarthric speech samples with varying intelligibility. *Journal of Speech and Hearing Research, 34,* 285–293.

Shewan, C. (1980). *Auditory Comprehension Test for Sentences.* Chicago: Biolinguistics Clinical Institute.

Shewan, C. (1988). The Shewan spontaneous language analysis (SSLA) system for aphasic adults: Description, reliability, and validity. *Journal of Communication Disorders, 21,* 103–138.

Shewan, C., & Bandur, D. (1986). *Treatment of aphasia: A language-oriented approach.* San Diego, CA: College Hill Press.

Shewan, C., & Kertesz, A. (1984). Effects of speech and language treatment on recovery from aphasia. *Brain & Language, 23,* 272–299.

Shuttleworth, E., & Huber, S. (1988). The naming disorder of dementia of Alzheimer type. *Brain & Language, 34,* 222–234.

Silver, L., & Halpern, H. (1992). Word-finding abilities of three types of aphasic subjects. *Journal of Psycholinguistic Research, 21*, 317–348.

Silverman, F. (1989). *Communication for the speechless.* Englewood Cliffs, NJ: Prentice-Hall.

Simmons, N. (1983). Acoustic analysis of ataxic dysarthria: An approach to monitoring treatment. In W. Berry (Ed.), *Clinical dysarthria* (pp. 283–294). San Diego, CA: College Hill Press.

Simpson, M., Till, J., & Goff, A. (1988). Long term treatment of severe dysarthria. *Journal of Speech and Hearing Disorders, 53*, 433–440.

Skenes, L., & Trullinger, R. (1988). Error patterns during repetition of consonant-vowel-consonant syllables by apraxic speakers. *Journal of Communication Disorders, 21*, 263–269.

Sklar, M. (1973). *Sklar Aphasia Scale.* Los Angeles: Western Psychological Services.

Smith, S., Murdoch, B., & Chenery, H. (1989). Semantic abilities in dementia of the Alzheimer's type. *Brain & Language, 36*, 314–324.

Sohlberg, M., & Ehlhardt, L. (1998). Case report: Management of confabulation after subarachnoid hemorrhage. *Neurophysiology and neurogenic speech and language disorders, 8*(2) [Special Interest Division Newsletter; Rockville, MD: American Speech-Language-Hearing Association].

Sohlberg, M., & Mateer, C. (1989). *Introduction to cognitive rehabilitation: Theory and practice.* New York: Guilford Press.

Solomon, N., & Hixon, T. (1993). Speech breathing in Parkinson's disease. *Journal of Speech and Hearing Research, 36*, 294–310.

Solomon, N., & Stierwalt, J. (1995). Strength and endurance training for dysarthria. *Neurophysiology and neurogenic speech & language disorders, 5*(4) [Special Interest Division Newsletter; Rockville, MD: American Speech-Language-Hearing Association].

Sparks, R., & Deck, J. (1994). Melodic intonation therapy. In R. Chapey (Ed.), *Language intervention strategies in adult aphasia* (pp. 368–379). Baltimore: Williams & Wilkins.

Sparks, R., & Holland, A. (1976). Method: Melodic intonation therapy for aphasia. *Journal of Speech and Hearing Disorders, 41*, 287–297.

Spreen, O., & Benton, A. (1969). *Neurosensory center comprehensive examination for aphasia.* Victoria, Canada: University of Victoria Neuropsychology Laboratory.

Spreen, O., & Risser, A. (1991). Assessment of aphasia. In M. Sarno (Ed.), *Acquired aphasia* (pp. 73–150). New York: Academic Press.

Square, P. (1981). *Auditory perceptual abilities of patients with apraxia of speech.* Unpublished doctoral dissertation, Kent State University, Kent, OH.

Square, P., & Martin, R. (1994). The nature and treatment of neuromotor speech disorders in aphasia. In R. Chapey (Ed.), *Language intervention strategies in adult aphasia* (pp. 467–498). Baltimore: Williams & Wilkins.

Square-Storer, P., Darley, F., & Sommers, R. (1988). Nonspeech and speech processing skills in patients with aphasia and apraxia of speech. *Brain & Language, 33,* 65–85.

Square-Storer, P., & Hayden, D. (1989). Prompt treatment. In P. Square-Storer (Ed.), *Acquired apraxia of speech in aphasic adults* (pp. 190–219). London: Erlbaum.

Stemmer, B., Giroux, F., & Joanette, Y. (1994). Production and evaluation of requests by right hemisphere brain-damaged individuals. *Brain & Language, 47,* 1–31.

Stengel, E. (1964). Speech disorders and mental disorders. In A. DeReuck & M. O'Connor (Eds.), *Disorders of language* (pp. 285–292). London: Churchill.

Stevens, E. (1989). Multiple input phoneme therapy. In P. Square-Storer (Ed.), *Acquired apraxia of speech in aphasic adults* (pp. 220–238). London: Erlbaum.

St. Louis, K., & Ruscello, D. (1987). *Oral Speech Mechanism Screening Examination* (rev. ed.). Austin, TX: PRO-ED.

Strand, E., & McNeil, M. (1996). Effects of length and linguistic complexity on temporal acoustic measures in apraxia of speech. *Journal of Speech and Hearing Research, 39,* 1018–1033.

Swindell, C., & Hammons, J. (1991). Poststroke depression: Neurologic, physiologic, diagnostic, and treatment implications. *Journal of Speech and Hearing Research, 34,* 325–333.

Swindell, C., Holland, A., Fromm, D., & Greenhouse, J. (1988). Characteristics of recovery of drawing ability in left and right brain-damaged patients. *Brain and Cognition, 7*, 16–30.

Swindell, C., Holland, A., & Reinmuth, O. (1998). Aphasia and related adult disorders. In G. Shames, E. Wiig, & W. Secord (Eds.), *Human communication disorders: An introduction* (pp. 472–509). Needham Heights, MA: Allyn & Bacon.

Taber's cyclopedic medical dictionary (18th ed.). (1997). Philadelphia: F. A. Davis.

Thompson, C., Shapiro, L., Roberts, M. (1993). Treatment of sentence production deficits in aphasia: A linguistic-specific approach to wh- interrogative training and generalization. *Aphasiology, 7*, 111–133.

Tikofsky, R., & Tikofsky, R. (1964). Intelligibility measures of dysarthric speech. *Journal of Speech and Hearing Research, 7*, 325–333.

Tomoeda, C., Bayles, K., & Boone, D. (1990). Speech rate and syntactic complexity effects in the auditory comprehension of Alzheimer patients. *Journal of Communication Disorders, 23*, 151–190.

Tompkins, C. (1990). Knowledge and strategies for processing lexical metaphor after right or left hemisphere brain damage. *Journal of Speech & Hearing Research, 33*, 307–316.

Tompkins, C. (1991a). Automatic and effortful processing of emotional intonation after right or left brain damage. *Journal of Speech and Hearing Research, 34*, 820–830.

Tompkins, C. (1991b). Redundancy enhances emotional inferencing by right- and left-hemisphere damaged adults. *Journal of Speech and Hearing Research, 34*, 1142–1149.

Tompkins, C. (1995). *Right hemisphere communication disorders: Theory and management.* San Diego, CA: Singular Publishing Group.

Tompkins, C., Bloise, C., Timko, M., & Baumgartner, A. (1994). Working memory and inference revision in brain-damaged and normally aging adults. *Journal of Speech & Hearing Research, 37*, 896–912.

Tompkins, C., Boada, R., & McGarry, K. (1992). The access and processing of familiar idioms by brain-damaged and normally aging adults. *Journal of Speech & Hearing Research, 35,* 626–637.

Tompkins, C., & Flowers, C. (1985). Perception of emotional intonation by brain-damaged adults: The influence of task processing levels. *Journal of Speech and Hearing Research, 28,* 527–538.

Tompkins, C., Holland, A., Ratcliff, G., Costello, A., Leahy, L., & Cowell, V. (1990). Predicting cognitive recovery from closed-head-injury in children and adolescents. *Brain & Cognition, 13,* 86–97.

Tompkins, C., Marshall, R., & Phillips, D. (1980). Aphasic patients in a rehabilitation program: Scheduling speech and language services. *Archives of Physical Medicine and Rehabilitation, 66,* 252–257.

Towne, R., & Banick, P. (1989). The effect of stimulus color on naming performance of aphasic adults. *Journal of Communication Disorders, 22,* 397–405.

Towne, R., & Crary, M. (1988). Verbal reaction time patterns in aphasic adults: Consideration for apraxia of speech. *Brain & Language, 35,* 138–153.

Trost, J. (1970). *Patterns of articulatory deficits in patients with Broca's aphasia.* Unpublished doctoral dissertation, Northwestern University, Chicago.

Trost, J., & Canter, G. (1974). Apraxia of speech in patients with Broca's aphasia: A study of phonemic production accuracy and error patterns. *Brain & Language, 1,* 63–79.

Tseng, C., McNeil, M., & Molenkovic, P. (1993). An investigation of attention allocation deficits in aphasia. *Brain & Language, 45,* 276–296.

Turner, G., Tjaden, K., & Weismer, G. (1995). The influence of speaking rate on vowel and speech intelligibility for individuals with amyotrophic lateral sclerosis. *Journal of Speech and Hearing Research, 38,* 1001–1013.

Turner, G., & Weismer, G. (1993). Characteristics of speaking rate in the dysarthria associated with amyotrophic lateral sclerosis. *Journal of Speech and Hearing Research, 36,* 1134–1144.

Ulatowska, H., Freedman-Stern, R., Doyel, A., & Macaluso-Haynes, S. (1983). Production of narrative discourse in aphasia. *Brain & Language, 19,* 317–334.

Vanhalle, C., Van der Linden, M., Belleville, S., & Gilbert, B. (1998). Putting names on faces: Use of a spaced retrieval strategy in a patient with dementia of the Alzheimer type. *Neurophysiology and neurogenic speech and language disorders, 8*(4) [Special Interest Division Newsletter; Rockville, MD: American Speech-Language-Hearing Association].

Van Lancker, D., & Klein, K. (1990). Preserved recognition of familiar personal names in global aphasia. *Brain & Language, 39,* 511–529.

Vignolo, L. (1964). Evolution of aphasia and language rehabilitation: A retrospective exploratory study. *Cortex, 1,* 344–367.

Volin, R., Goldfarb, R., Raphael, L., & Weinstein, B. (1990). Language, speech and hearing in Pick's disease: A case study. *Clinical Gerontologist, 10,* 93–98.

Wagenaar, E., Snow, C., & Prins, R. (1975). Spontaneous speech of aphasic patients: A psycholinguistic analysis. *Brain & Language, 2,* 281–303.

Wallace, G., & Canter, G. (1985). Effects of personally relevant language materials on the performance of severely aphasic individuals. *Journal of Speech and Hearing Disorders, 50,* 385–390.

Wambaugh, J., Kalinyak-Flisger, M., West, J., & Doyle, P. (1998). Effects of treatment for sound errors in apraxia of speech and aphasia. *Journal of Speech-Language-Hearing Research, 41,* 725–743.

Warren, R. (1977). Rehearsal for naming in apraxia of speech. In R. Brookshire (Ed.), *Clinical aphasiology: Conference proceedings* (pp. 80–90). Minneapolis, MN: BRK Publishers.

Watterson, T., McFarlane, S., & Menicucci, A. (1990). Vibratory characteristics of teflon-injected and noninjected paralyzed vocal folds. *Journal of Speech and Hearing Disorders, 55,* 61–66.

Webster, D. (1999). *Neuroscience of communication.* San Diego, CA: Singular.

Wechsler, D. (1981). *Wechsler Adult Intelligence Scale–Revised Manual.* New York: Psychological Corp.

Weinstein, E., Lyerly, O., Cole, M., & Ozer, M. (1966). Meaning in jargon aphasia. *Cortex, 2*, 165–187.

Weisenburg, T., & McBride, K. (1935). *Aphasia.* New York: Hafner.

Wepman, J. (1951). *Recovery from aphasia.* New York: Ronald Press.

Wepman, J., & Jones, L. (1961). *The language modalities test for aphasia.* Chicago: Education Industry Service.

Wernicke, C. (1874). *Das Aphasische Symptomenkomplex* [*The aphasia symptom complex*]. Breslau, Germany: Cohn & Weigart.

Wertz, R. (1984). Response to treatment in patients with apraxia of speech. In J. Rosenbek, M. McNeil, & A. Aronson (Eds.), *Apraxia of speech: Physiology, acoustics, linguistics, management* (pp. 257–276). San Diego, CA: College Hill Press.

Wertz, R. (1985). Neuropathologies of speech and language: An introduction to patient management. In D. F. Johns (Ed.), *Clinical management of neurogenic communicative disorders* (pp. 1–96). Boston: Little, Brown.

Wertz, R. (1992). A single case for group treatment studies in aphasia. In *Aphasia treatment: Current approaches and research opportunities* (NIH Publication No. 93-3424). Bethesda, MD: NIH.

Wertz, R., Collins, M., Weiss, D., Kurtzke, J., Friden, T., Brookshire, R., Pierce, J., Holtzapple, P., Hubbard, D., Porch, B., West, J., Davis, L., Matovich, V., Morley, G., & Resurreccion, E. (1981). Veterans administration cooperative study in aphasia: A comparison of individual and group treatment. *Journal of Speech and Hearing Research, 24*, 580–594.

Wertz, R., LaPointe, L., & Rosenbek, J. (1984). *Apraxia of speech in adults.* New York: Grune & Stratton.

Wertz, R., Weiss, D., Aten, J., Brookshire, R., Garcia-Bunuel, L., Holland, A., Kurtzke, J., LaPointe, L., Milianti, F., Brannegan, R., Greenbaum, H., Marshall, R., Vogel, D., Carter, J., Barnes, N., & Goodman, R. (1986). A comparison of clinic, home, and deferred language treatment for aphasia: A VA cooperative study. *Archives of Neurology, 43*, 653–658.

Wiegersma, S., Post, H., Veldhuijsen, M., & DeVries, L. (1988). Encoding of frequency of occurrence by aphasia patients: Attentional or linguistic defects. *Cortex, 24,* 433–441.

Wilson, R., Kazniak, A., Bacon, L., Fox, J., & Kelly, M. (1982). Facial recognition memory in dementia. *Cortex, 18,* 329–336.

Winner, E., Brownell, H., Happe, F., Blum, A., & Pincus, D. (1998). Distinguishing lies from jokes: Theory of mind deficits and discourse interpretation in right-hemisphere brain-damaged patients. *Brain and Language, 62,* 89–106.

Wit, J., Maassen, B., Gabreels, F., & Thoonen, G. (1993). Maximum performance tests in children with developmental spastic dysarthria. *Journal of Speech and Hearing Research, 36,* 452–459.

Wolk, L. (1986). Marked analysis of consonant error productions in apraxia of speech. *Journal of Communication Disorders, 19,* 133–160.

Wood, L., Hughes, J., Hayes, K., & Wolfe, D. (1992). Reliability of labial closure force measurements in normal subjects and patients with CNS disorders. *Journal of Speech and Hearing Research, 25,* 252–258.

Ylvisaker, M., & Feeney, T. (1998). A Vygotskyan approach to rehabilitation after TBI: A case illustration. *Neurophysiology and neurogenic speech and language disorders, 8*(2) [Special Interest Division Newsletter; Rockville, MD: American Speech-Hearing-Language Association].

Ylvisaker, M., & Szekeres, S. (1994). Communication disorders associated with closed head injury. In R. Chapey (Ed.), *Language intervention strategies in adult aphasia* (pp. 546–567). Baltimore: Williams & Wilkins.

Yorkston, K. (1996). Treatment efficacy: Dysarthria. *Journal of Speech and Hearing Research, 39,* S46–S57.

Yorkston, K., & Beukelman, D. (1980a). An analysis of connected speech samples of aphasic and normal speakers. *Journal of Speech and Hearing Disorders, 45,* 27–36.

Yorkston, K., & Beukelman, D. (1980b). A clinician-judged technique for quantifying dysarthric speech based on single-word intelligibility. *Journal of Communication Disorders, 13,* 15–31.

Yorkston, K., & Beukelman, D. (1981a). *Assessment of Intelligibility of Dysarthric Speech.* Tigard, OR: CC Publications.

Yorkston, K., & Beukelman, D. (1981b). Communication efficiency of dysarthric speakers as measured by sentence intelligibility and speaking rate. *Journal of Speech and Hearing Disorders, 46,* 296–301.

Yorkston, K., & Beukelman, D. (1983). The influence of judge familiarization with the speaker on dysarthric speech intelligibility. In W. Berry (Ed.), *Clinical dysarthria* (pp. 153–163). San Diego, CA: College Hill Press.

Yorkston, K., Beukelman, D., & Bell, K. (1988). *Clinical management of dysarthric speakers.* San Diego, CA: College Hill Press.

Yorkston, K., Beukelman, D., & Honsinger, M. (1989). Perceived articulatory adequacy and velopharyngeal function in dysarthric speakers. *Archives of Physical Medicine and Rehabilitation, 70,* 313–317.

Yorkston, K., Hammen, V., Beukelman, D., & Traynor, C. (1990). The effect of rate control on the intelligibility and naturalness of dysarthric speech. *Journal of Speech and Hearing Disorders, 55,* 550–560.

Yorkston, K., Strand, E., & Kennedy, M. (1996). Comprehensibility of dysarthric speech: Implications for assessment and treatment planning. *American Journal of Speech-Language Pathology, 5,* 55–66.

Yoss, K., & Darley, F. (1974). Therapy in developmental apraxia of speech. *Language, Speech and Hearing Services in the Schools, 5,* 23–31.

Zemlin, W. (1998). *Speech and hearing science: Anatomy and physiology.* Needham Heights, MA: Allyn & Bacon.

Ziegler, W., Hartmann, E., & Hoople, P. (1993). Syllabic timing in dysarthria. *Journal of Speech and Hearing Research, 36,* 683–693.

Ziegler, W., & von Cramon, D. (1986). Spastic dysarthria after acquired brain injury: An acoustic study. *British Journal of Disorders of Communication, 21,* 173–187.

Zraick, R., & Boone, D. (1991). Spouse attitudes toward the person with aphasia. *Journal of Speech and Hearing Research, 34,* 123–128.

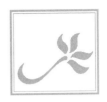

Index

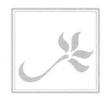

About the Author

Harvey Halpern is a professor in the Department of Linguistics and Communication Disorders at Queens College and on the doctoral faculty in the Program in Speech and Hearing Sciences at the Graduate Center of the City University of New York.

He has worked as a speech–language pathologist at the Brooklyn College Speech and Hearing Center, for the New York City Board of Education, and in private practice. In addition to his above-mentioned teaching position, he is currently involved in a part-time private practice.

He has published numerous articles, several chapters, and is Editor of the PRO-ED series *Studies in Communicative Disorders,* to which he contributed *Adult Aphasia* (1972) and *Language and Motor Speech Disorders in Adults* (1986). He has participated in many professional panels, including delivering a number of short courses. He was a post-doctoral fellow at the Mayo Clinic and is a member of both the Academy of Aphasia and the Academy of Neurologic Communication Disorders and Sciences.

He is a member with licensure in speech–language pathology and a past president of the New York State Speech-Language-Hearing Association. He is a member with certification in speech–language pathology, a former legislative councilor, and a fellow in the American Speech-Language-Hearing Association.

29
Speed Sample